*The Five-Factor Model
of Personality*

The Five-Factor Model of Personality
THEORETICAL PERSPECTIVES

Edited by
JERRY S. WIGGINS

THE GUILFORD PRESS
New York London

© 1996 The Guilford Press
A Division of Guilford Publications, Inc.
72 Spring Street, New York, NY 10012

Printed in the United States of America

This book is printed on acid-free paper.

Last digit is print number: 9 8 7 6 5 4 3 2 1

Library of Congress Cataloging-in-Publication Data available from
the Publisher

ISBN 1-57230-068-X

Contributors

David M. Buss, Ph.D., Department of Psychology, University of Michigan, Ann Arbor, Michigan

Paul T. Costa, Jr., Ph.D., Laboratory of Personality and Cognition, National Institute on Aging, National Institutes of Health, Baltimore, Maryland

John M. Digman, Ph.D., Oregon Research Institute, Eugene, Oregon

Lewis R. Goldberg, Ph.D., Department of Psychology, University of Oregon, and Oregon Research Institute, Eugene, Oregon

Robert Hogan, Ph.D., Department of Psychology, University of Tulsa, Tulsa, Oklahoma

Robert R. McCrae, Ph.D., Personality, Stress, and Coping Section, Gerontology Research Center, National Institute on Aging, National Institutes óf Health, Baltimore, Maryland

Gerard Saucier, Ph.D., Department of Psychology, California State University–San Bernardino, San Bernardino, California

Paul D. Trapnell, Ph.D., Department of Psychology, University of British Columbia, Vancouver, British Columbia, Canada

Jerry S. Wiggins, Ph.D., Department of Psychology, University of British Columbia, Vancouver, British Columbia, Canada

Preface

There are many ways to define personality (as there should be), but I have always favored the rather loose, but encompassing, characterization of personality as the general psychology of individual differences. Such a definition is reflexive, in the Kellyian sense, because it may also be applied to differences among *investigators* in the ways in which they construe personality. The present volume could be viewed as a study of individual differences because it holds a stimulus constant (five-factor model of personality) and allows responses to vary freely. No respectable journal would accept this as a proper experiment, however, because the "subjects" were not selected randomly, nor could they be considered representative of an unselected population. More tellingly, the design of the study was biased by its exclusion of subjects who held contrary views about the value of the stimulus materials (e.g., Block, 1995; Eysenck, 1992; Hough, 1992; McAdams, 1992; Pervin, 1994; Tellegen, 1993; Waller & Ben-Porath, 1987). A few words of justification are clearly in order.

In an earlier climate of opinion, it was possible to offer a detailed and approving discussion of "a systematic and cumulative series of investigations of the structure of peer ratings" without giving offense (Wiggins, 1973, p. 339). Admittedly, the discussion just cited was relatively free of hyperbole (e.g., "*the* five-factor model"; "*Big* Five") and did not delimit alternatives (e.g., "plus or minus *two*"), nor did the narrative tone suggest "unabashed hubris" (McAdams, 1992). Such excesses of enthusiasm are more prevalent today and they have given rise, in some quarters, to serious concerns about a "big five bandwagon" (Waller & Ben-Porath, 1987) that has been "vigorously pursued and promoted" by its "boosters," "advocates," and "adherents" (Block, 1995).

It is perhaps not accidental that the contributors to the present volume include just those investigators who have been most fre-

vii

quently accused of enthusiastic advocacy; but the *intent* of this collection of essays is neither subversive nor defensive. Instead, these essays are meant to illustrate (1) the diversity of theoretical perspectives that are currently being brought to bear on the five-factor model (FFM) of personality and (2) the opportunities the FFM can provide for communication and the sharing of ideas among some of the major figures in contemporary personality research, investigators whose subdisciplinary "boundaries" might otherwise have proven less permeable to such exchanges.

With respect to the first purpose of this collection, I must admit that of all the criticisms leveled at the FFM, the charge that this body of research is "atheoretical" has struck me as the most unfair. The present collection of essays should make clear that there are indeed well-articulated theoretical perspectives being brought to bear on the FFM and that they do *not* stem from a monolithic world view. Instead, the diverse perspectives on the FFM provided by the lexical theory (Saucier & Goldberg, Chapter 2), trait theory (McCrae & Costa, Chapter 3), interpersonal theory (Wiggins & Trapnell, Chapter 4), socioanalytic theory (Hogan, Chapter 5), and evolutionary theory (Buss, Chapter 6) offer a wide choice of attractive bandwagons to those who are inclined toward jumping.

As to the second purpose, it should be evident that the contributors are well acquainted with each other's work and that there are areas of agreement and disagreement among investigators from different subdisciplines. Being privy to the correspondence among contributors resulting from the circulation of draft copies and comments prior to publication, I am well aware that some of these disagreements are rather fundamental in nature—which only serves to underscore the erroneousness of the notion that there is a conceptual "party line" adhered to by the major contributors to research on the FFM. The *heuristic value* of the FFM may be illustrated by comparing the scope of topics covered in the present essays to those treated in the literature of personality structure of any other period within the last 20 years.

All contemporary research in personality has a history and the FFM has a particularly long and curious one. **John M. Digman** has been a major contributor to that history over the last 30 years and, because of the depth and breadth of his knowledge of the field, has in recent times become the unofficial "historian" of the FFM. The history of the FFM has been reiterated so many times that it has the status of a well-worn folk tale. But Digman's treatment of this topic in

Chapter 1 provides a truly fresh approach by drawing striking parallels with other sciences and by delving even more deeply into the origins of the model itself.

Although the lexical tradition in personality psychology is a longstanding one that includes milestone studies by such authors as Allport, Cattell, and Norman, the more recent work of **Lewis R. Goldberg** in this tradition has been so fundamental, so extensive, and so influential that it has become difficult to distinguish the subdiscipline from the person. In Chapter 2, **Gerard Saucier** and Goldberg provide a definitive statement of just what the lexical perspective is (and is not) and emphasize further the important differences between the "Big Five" model of the lexical tradition and the FFM of the psychometric–trait tradition. Although they eschew the use of the term "theoretical," the authors offer a host of alternative adjectives to characterize the position that provides the linguistic foundations for the FFM.

Robert R. McCrae and **Paul T. Costa, Jr.**, in the course of their "astonishingly fruitful research collaboration" (Block, 1995), have immeasurably enriched the nomological network surrounding the FFM by their studies of the differing theoretical contexts and areas of application to which the model is applicable. In Chapter 3, they attempt to combine the conceptual insights of the classic theories of personality and contemporary research within a metatheoretical framework for "a new generation of personality theories." Within that framework, they sketch a theory, based on FFM research, as a "rough prototype" of the future theories they envision.

Jerry S. Wiggins has been a longstanding advocate of theory-driven personality assessment procedures in general and the interpersonal circumplex model in particular. In Chapter 6, Wiggins and **Paul D. Trapnell** provide the conceptual foundations for a dyadic–interactional perspective on the FFM that is guided by the metatheoretical concepts of agency and communion. This perspective assigns a conceptual priority to the first two factors of the model and emphasizes the manifestations of agentic and communal concerns within the remaining three factors.

In the course of his distinguished career as theorist, critic, and personality assessment practitioner, **Robert Hogan** has evolved an integrative theory of personality that stands in bold contrast to more traditional trait theories. As Hogan notes in Chapter 5, psychoanalytic and symbolic interactionist thought provide a radically different perspective on the FFM from that espoused by McCrae and Costa.

This chapter provides an especially clear introduction to the socioanalytic perspective and its implications for trait theory and measurement.

All of the chapters in this book place the FFM within the contexts of earlier theoretical perspectives, and the tradition of evolutionary theory is certainly among the most venerable of all traditions that might be covered. Although clearly in the Darwinian tradition, the evolutionary psychology that **David M. Buss** applies to the FFM in Chapter 6 is a very recent paradigm that is meant to serve as a metatheory for contemporary psychological science. During the last decade, Buss's persuasive arguments and ingenious empirical studies have brought this paradigm to the attention of a wide audience of scholars and general readers. Chapter 6 serves both as an introduction to the central evolutionary concept of *psychological mechanism* and as a most distinctive alternative perspective on the FFM.

The full-range of theoretical perspectives encompassed by these contributions may be appreciated with reference to the phenotypic–genotypic distinction made by Saucier and Goldberg in Chapter 2. Lexical research, such as that of Saucier and Goldberg, focuses on ordinary language descriptions of observed personality attributes (*phenotypes*) and does not attempt causal explanations of the phenomena described. In contrast, many trait theorists in the FFM tradition have focused on generative mechanisms (*genotypes*) that are postulated to underlie surface attributes, as exemplified by the evolutionary psychology approach of Buss in the final chapter. The contributions of McCrae and Costa, Wiggins and Trapnell, and Hogan have been ordered (roughly) along this continuum of relative emphasis on phenotypic and genotypic constructs.

Reading these conceptually rich essays may help one to place some of the current debates over the utility of the FFM in a somewhat broader context. For example, the frequent (and quite legitimate) questions that have been raised concerning the *number* of dimensions that is necessary and sufficient for a consensual working model take on additional meaning in the present context. As new dimensions are proposed, questions raised by different perspectives might be considered:

> To what extent is this dimension replicable across samples of subjects, targets of description, and variations in analytic procedures across different natural languages? (*lexical perspective:* Saucier & Goldberg)

How much does this dimension add to our prediction of characteristic adaptations to life circumstances? (*trait perspective:* McCrae & Costa)

To what extent does this dimension interfere with or facilitate agentic and communal enterprises within society? (*dyadic–interactional perspective:* Wiggins & Trapnell)

To what extent is this dimension weighted by observers in their evaluation of the potential social contributions of others? (*socioanalytic perspective:* Hogan)

How relevant is this dimension to solving social adaptive problems, such as the forming of strategic alliances and the avoidance of strategic interference? (*evolutionary perspective:* Buss)

JERRY S. WIGGINS

References

Block, J. (1995). A contrarian view of the five-factor approach to personality description. *Psychological Bulletin, 117,* 187–215.

Eysenck, H. J. (1992). Four ways five-factors are *not* basic. *Personality and Individual Differences, 6,* 667–673.

Hough, L. (1992). The "Big Five" personality variables—construct confusion: Description versus prediction. *Human Performance, 5,* 139–155.

McAdams, D. P. (1992). The five-factor model *in* personality: A critical appraisal. *Journal of Personality, 60,* 329–361.

Pervin, L. A. (1994). A critical analysis of current trait theory. *Psychological Inquiry, 5,* 103–113.

Tellegen, A. (1993). Folk concepts and psychological concepts of personality and personality disorder. *Psychological Inquiry, 4,* 122–130.

Waller, N. G., & Ben-Porath, Y. S. (1987). Is it time for clinical psychology to embrace the five-factor model of personality? *American Psychologist, 42,* 887–889.

Wiggins, J.S. (1973). *Personality and prediction: Principles of personality assessment.* Reading, MA: Addison-Wesley.

Contents

*The Five-Factor Model
of Personality*

The Curious History of the Five-Factor Model

JOHN M. DIGMAN

There is today a "new look" to the field of personality, one that has attracted the attention of many researchers and writers as a conceptual scheme for uniting a field that at times has appeared to be chaotic (Cronbach, 1970). This is the five-factor model (FFM), or "Big Five,"[1] which emerged from obscurity in the 1980s. There was scant mention of this model in the textbooks or in the journals until recently; thus, a reasonable conclusion would be that its sudden emergence represents one of those "breakthroughs" in science that quickly revolutionize a field. It is puzzling to learn, then, that the model made its first appearance over 60 years ago. Perhaps this was some obscure report from an unknown researcher? Hardly; the report came from a well known and highly respected scientist, no less than Louis Thurstone (1934), as part of his Presidential Address to the 1933 meeting of the American Psychological Association. Commenting on his factor analysis of 60 adjectives, used by subjects to rate well known acquaintances, he remarked with evident surprise that, "It is of considerable psychological interest to know that the whole list of sixty adjectives can be accounted for by postulating only five independent common factors" (p. 13). However, as Goldberg (1993) has noted, Thurstone failed to follow up on what might have been the launching of the Big Five model in the mid-1930s, turning his attention instead to the development of a questionnaire, the Thurstone Temperament Schedule. His thought-provoking conclusions, printed prominently in the *Psychological Review* and presumably at least noted by any psychologist interested in the study of individual differences, failed to generate any further investigation.

Other Early Harbingers

Webb and Garnett

Enlarging on the earlier work of Spearman (1904) and his General Factor (g) of intelligence, Webb (1915) analyzed instructors' ratings of two groups of male students, one in their early 20s, the other with an average age of 12. The students were rated with respect to 48 characteristics, some of which were suggestive of g, whereas others reflected "moral characteristics." Webb found the g factor, as expected. He also noted a second factor that was something quite different from g. This was indicated by such characteristics as "Tendency not to abandon tasks," "Perseverence in the face of obstacles," and "Conscientiousness." Webb interpreted this as Will, for which he proposed the symbol w.

Later, Garnett (1919) analyzed Webb's correlations further and concluded that a third factor could be isolated from the data. Garnett interpreted this new factor as *Cleverness*. This interpretation immediately suggests the Intellect (Openness) factor of the Big Five. However, a close perusal of the variables that correlated most highly with this factor suggests to the modern reader that Garnett was wide of the mark, when he proposed the term "Cleverness" for this dimension; Garnett's Cleverness is clearly Extraversion, indicated by "General tendency to be cheerful," "Degree of sense of humour," "Fondness for large social gatherings," and "Wideness of his influence."

And so, by 1919, one finds evidence in the literature for three broad factors accounting for individual differences, Intellect (g), Conscientiousness (w), and Extraversion (c), to give the Webb–Garnett factors their current names. I can almost hear some objections to my interpretation of Webb's g as Intellect. However, it must be remembered that the characteristics that suggested Spearman's g to Webb were not paper-and-pencil test items in the measurement domain that Cattell (1957) has called T-data; rather, they were *ratings* of students by instructors, what Cattell has termed Life Record (L-data), based on the behavior record as observed by raters.

Moving a Bit Closer:
Four Nonintellective Temperament Dimensions

In 1933 a young protégé of Spearman, Raymond Cattell, published an analysis of a set of "temperament" traits, that is, non-intellective traits that are theoretically independent of the Spearman g factor. Using a set of 46 bipolar rating scales, 62 male college students rated other students well known to them. Each bipolar scale was defined in terms of brief descriptive phrases. For example, the rating scale "Good-Natured–Malicious" appeared as:

Good-Natured	Malicious
Generous. Well-wishing. Enjoys others' success. Good-natured in sense of being more ready to give than to take in small things. Not necessarily prepared for great or heroic self-sacrifice and unselfishness.	Cruel. Laughter sardonic. Disparages others. Inclined to be interested in and to enjoy others' misfortunes.

Like Webb and Garnett before him, Cattell (1933) noted a w factor, indicated by such characteristics as conscientious–unreliable, persistent–changeable, and persevering–willfully changeable, terms that strongly point to the Conscientiousness factor of the Big Five. Cattell also noted the Garnett c factor, for which he suggested the term *Surgency*, the first time this interpretation appears in the literature, and a Maturity factor, m, indicated by mature–willful, good-natured–malicious, and kind on principle–absence of kindness, items that can only be taken as indicants of the Agreeableness dimension of the Big Five.

Finally, there was a fourth factor, denoted by such terms as emotional–unemotional, balanced–extreme, objective–subjective, and frank–secretive, which, Cattell noted, "underlies a set of qualities which in clinical practice are commonly regarded as characterizing the well-adjusted rather than the maladjusted individual" (p. 323). Since "temperament" traits denoted the nonintellective aspects of individual differences, these four factors, to which Cattell doubtless would have added the Spearman g factor as a broad factor of intellect, may be regarded as the first glimpse of the Big Five. A comparison with Thurstone's (1934) five-factor solution indicates that Cattell's solution was closer to the contemporary model; Thurstone found five factors, but the content of these factors was rather different from the content of the Big Five.

In the mid-1930s, attention turned to personality questionnaires, and Guilford and Guilford (1936) applied the new Thurstone centroid method of factor analysis to 36 questionnaire type items (e.g., "Are your feelings rather easily hurt?"). The analysis found five factors, as indicated by trivial residuals following extraction of the fifth. The factors were identified as simply *S*, *E*, and *M*, although it seemed evident to the Guilfords that Factor *S* had a social flavor, *E* suggested emotion, and *M* was virtually a specific factor that was mostly related to the question "Are you a male?" Two other factors were difficult to interpret: One was indicated by sensitivity to others' feelings, carelessness of dress, impulsiveness, and daydreaming. The authors interpreted this as *Rhathymia* (R), a Greek word meaning freedom from care. The last factor, involving an interest in intellectual matters and liking to study the motives of others, suggested a "liking for thinking." Although inclined to see this as an aspect of introversion—that is, Thinking Introversion—the Guilfords cautiously labeled this simply as a "*T* factor." In terms of today's Big Five, it is possible to see four of these five factors as Extraversion (*S*), Emotional *In*stability (*E*), (lack of) Conscientiousness (with perhaps a bit of *Dis*agreeableness) (*R*), and Intellect (*T*). Looking over the Guilford questionnaire items, one can find only one question that would obviously suggest Agreeableness: "Are you inclined to be considerate of other people's feelings?" Consequently, because the analysis was based on what the variables had in common (i.e., a common factor analysis), Agreeableness could not have made its appearance in this study.

Three years later, Guilford and Guilford (1939) reported an analysis of an extended list of 89 questionnaire items, although only 30 of these were actually involved in the analysis. Nine centroid factors were extracted and rotated to an oblique solution by graphical means. Of these, only five could be clearly interpreted: Depression (*D*), Rhathymia (*R*), Liking for Thinking (*LT*), Shyness (*S*), and Thinking (*T*), which are suggestive of Emotional *In*stability, (Low) Conscientiousness, Intellect (both *LT* and *T*), and Introversion. Again, Agreeableness did not appear as a factor, having been represented, as before, only by the item regarding consideration for others' feelings.

The work of the Guilfords, then, went beyond the earlier work of the English group of investigators (Webb, Garnett, and Cattell), but only to the extent of finding a factor clearly related to Emotional Stability, a rather obvious personality dimension. From today's perspective, we may question the choice of items that were selected from the full list of 87 items for the analysis, but a factor analysis of an 87-variable correlation matrix was out of the question in those days.

Thus, by the 1940s, we were tantalizingly close to something like today's five-factor model. Had there been a conference attended by Webb, Garnett, the Guilfords, and Cattell, there might have been agreement on Extraversion (Garnett, Cattell, and the Guilfords), Conscientiousness (Webb, Garnett, Cattell, and the Guilfords), Emotional Stability (the Guilfords, and, very likely, Cattell), and Intellect (Webb, Garnett, Cattell, and the Guilfords). Considering the difficulty factor analysts have always had with finding appropriate labels for their factors, one might reasonably assume that much of the discussion would have centered on the interpretations of these four factors. However, all of these investigators might have agreed that the realm of individual differences, when surveyed by factor analysis, suggested somewhere around five factors.

Would anyone have questioned the absence of something like *aggression* or *love* from the list of factors, considering the widespread interest in psychoanalysis at that time? Would there have been doubts about a model of individual differences in terms of only four or five factors? And perhaps most instructive of all, were these two groups of investigators, both of whom relied on factor analysis as an analytic tool, at all aware of the relevance of what the other group was doing? An examination of the references cited by American authors of inventories during the period 1930–1950 leads one to conclude that there was little interchange of ideas across the Atlantic at this time, with the notable exception of Cattell, who brought his views and methods from England upon his move to the United States in 1937.

Cattell's Later Studies

In the mid-1940s, Cattell began an ambitious program of systematic research on personality traits, based on the compendium of personality trait terms assembled by Allport and Odbert (1936). It is difficult to feel anything other than admiration for this pioneer researcher, who like the Guilfords, would seriously consider a factor analysis of 35 bipolar scales, based on peer ratings of 373 male university students. The clerical labor involved, using the clumsy calculators of that time, was monumental, enough to dampen anyone's enthusiasm for such an undertaking. Nonetheless, Cattell (1944) forged ahead, apparently influenced by early drafts of what was to become the definitive treatment of factor analysis for many researchers—Thurstone's *Multiple Factor Analysis* (1947). As Cattell (1947) subsequently put it, "We planned to proceed by Thurstone's practice of removing a probable excess of factors, deciding thereafter the true number by the verdict of how many could be reduced to residuals in the process of rotation"(p. 206). The principle to which Cattell referred can be found in Thurstone's text: "It is a safe rule to continue the factoring until one is sure that the factoring has gone far enough. *Too many factors can do no harm*" (p. 509, italics added). This was a fateful principle for both Thurstone and Cattell. Employing this principle as a guide, Cattell removed 12 factors from the correlations among his 35 rating variables. Following rotation, which was guided by the Thurstone principle of simple structure, Cattell offered interpretations for these factors, albeit with some diffidence regarding several of them. Soon thereafter, Cattell (1947) completed another study, based like the first on men only, and concluded that "nine of the 11 factors . . . are exactly identifiable with those of the earlier study" (p. 217). A third study, based on women (Cattell, 1948), found 11 factors, some of them apparent replicates from the male studies, others new. On the basis of these three studies, including the factors that did not replicate but were "new factors," Cattell put all three results together to develop his 16 PF (Sixteen Personality Factors) Questionnaire.

I have reviewed these studies elsewhere (Digman & Takemoto-Chock, 1981) and found them troubling in several aspects. First, there were far too many factors extracted by today's standards (Goldberg & Digman, 1994). In addition, an examination of the correlation matrix of the female sample (with correction in sign for one correlation and with deletion of a college aptitude variable that correlated little with the 35 rating variables) might suggest five or six factors to someone today, inasmuch as the eigenvalues become less than unity after the sixth and trivial ($< .70$) after the seventh. Many of Cattell's factors were not well defined: Factor L in the first study, for example, had one item with a loading of .22 and all others with loadings between .16 and .19. Factor N in the third study, indicated by two variables with communalities in excess of unity, should have been an indication that something was seriously wrong. There was—the correlation for the two principal variables denoting this factor had been entered into the analysis with the wrong sign.

Ironically, Cattell's third study (the women's study) provided an excellent Big Five solution (Digman & Takemoto-Chock, 1981).

When the sign for the correlation of the variables defining Factor *N* was corrected, there was no evidence for anything beyond seven factors, and a five-factor solution provided a remarkably good match with other five-factor solutions. Four of the factors were good matches for the four isolated previously by Cattell (1933) in his temperament study; the fifth, indicated by only two items, was vaguely suggestive of the Openness interpretation of Factor V (Costa & McCrae, 1985). Cattell, then, had he built upon the foundation of his earlier temperament study, might have been the first to note the Big Five, for they were clearly present in his data.

Reflecting later on these early studies, Cattell (1950) believed that "only six—*A, B, F, H, K,* and *M*—are repeatedly confirmed" (p. 57). Nonetheless, these and other minor—and nonreplicable factors—made their way into the 16 PF and into most of the textbooks as an example of the "factor approach" to personality.

Fiske's Analyses of 22 Rating Scales

In 1947, Donald Fiske began a year-long analysis of three sets of correlations based on 22 of Cattell's rating scales. By the time he had removed five factors, little of the original correlations remained. Using graphical rotation and an oblique solution, Fiske (1949) identified his five factors as "Social Adaptability," "Conformity," "Emotional Control," "Inquiring Intellect," and "Confident Self-Expression." On the basis of the scales defining these factors, the first four may be recognized as today's Extraversion, Agreeableness, Emotional Stability, and Intellect (Fiske's "Inquiring Intellect" is still one of the best labels for this dimension). The fifth factor was "not as clear-cut as those previously discussed" (p. 338). From today's vantage point, it appears to be a second Extraversion factor, incorporating some of the Extraversion variables not in Factor 1. Missing from this list is Conscientiousness, although Digman and Takemoto-Chock (1981) in their reanalysis of Fiske's study, found evidence for this dimension, particularly from the "staff ratings data," indicated by such Conscientious markers as conscientious–not conscientious, serious–frivolous, and predictable–unpredictable.

Fiske (D. W. Fiske, personal communication, August 25, 1994) was not concerned by the much simpler solution he achieved, as compared with that of Cattell. Rather, he was pleased to find that his five-factor solution appeared to be relatively stable across three different sources—self-ratings, peer ratings, and supervisors' ratings. Fiske reported his findings in a well regarded journal that enjoyed a wide readership among research psychologists in the fields of social psychology and personality. Today, it strikes one as quite odd that it was almost completely ignored: Here was a carefully done study, carried out scrupulously under excellent conditions, and with results that were stable across three modes of data gathering, a stability of results not to be seen again for more than a decade. Much later, a reanalysis of Fiske's correlations (Digman & Takemoto-Chock, 1981), confirmed the essential correctness of Fiske's analyses. The correspondence of a five-factor solution with current views of the meaning of the Big Five was striking. As far as I have been able to determine, the results of this excellent study by Fiske did not appear in any personality textbook until the publication of Wiggins (1973) influential graduate-level text on assessment.

Thurstone's Study of Temperament

Having found a five-factor solution for peer ratings in the early 1930s, Thurstone, after spending years developing factor techniques, culminating in the definitive text, *Multiple Factor Analysis* (Thurstone, 1947), turned his attention again to the study of the temperament (i.e., nonintellective) aspects of personality. A study by Lovell (1945) had factored 13 personality scales designed by Guilford and his coworkers over the years (Guilford & Guilford, 1936, 1939a, 1939b). Thurstone (1951) analyzed Lovell's correlations, using what were then state-of-the-art methods—that is, as found in his own text. From the 13 variables, nine (!) factors were extracted and rotated by graphical means to simple structure. That nine factors should be extracted from the correlations of 13 variables hardly suggests parsimony, but Thurstone (1947), having urged others not to worry about overextraction, proceeded to extract factors until his last residual matrix contained minute values. Reanalysis of these correlations indicates that Thurstone was surely overextracting by any contemporary standard; the fifth eigenvalue of the full matrix is .97, but from the sixth to the ninth, the eigenvalues drop from .44 to .25. Thurstone interpreted seven of these nine factors as Reflective, Impulsive, Sociable, Active, Dominant, Vigorous, and Emotionally Stable, terms that have found their way into many personality texts. However, if a more contemporary analysis is done, in terms of five components with varimax rotation, four of the Big Five are clearly there, with Masculinity emerging as something of a specific dimension.[2] There is nothing of Conscientiousness in this analysis, as there is no suggestion of an Agreeableness factor in the Guilford and Guilford (1936) variables. Component 1 is clearly Extraversion, 2 is Agreeableness (indicated even with a test by that name), 3 is Emotional Stability, and 5 is most likely indicative of the domain of the Big Five dimension of Intellect.

The First Clear Appearances of the Big Five

The Conscientious Investigators: Tupes and Christal

More than a decade after the publication of Fiske's study, two U.S. Air Force researchers, Ernest Tupes and Raymond Christal (1961, 1992), using a set of 30 scales borrowed from Cattell's slightly larger list, found five factors that were stable across replications and in their reanalyses of Cattell's (1947, 1948) and Fiske's (1949) correlations. The study was in many ways a model factor analysis, as was a second study by Tupes and Kaplan (1961), which demonstrated the robustness of the five-factor solution, regardless of whether socially desirable or socially undesirable characteristics were analyzed. In addition, Tupes and Christal conducted what in essence may be seen as a meta-analysis, relating their own results to results obtained by analyzing the correlations of other investigators and comparing the factors across studies. It was unfortunate that the results of these studies were published as Air Force Technical Reports and thus were seen by few researchers of personality. Despite this obscurity, the report marks the beginning of a serious interest in the five-factor model, at least on the part of a few researchers.

The Observant Three: Norman, Borgatta, and Smith

One of these researchers was Warren Norman (1963b), who presented a five-factor solution of 20 peer rating scales at the 1963 meeting of the Society of Multivariate Experimental Psychology (Norman, 1963a). That five factors, based on the correlations of these 20 scales, might represent "an adequate taxonomy of personality attributes" (Norman, 1963b, p. 582), probably seemed simplistic to many personality investigators. Certainly, it did to me, for at the same meeting I had presented an analysis of child personality attributes as rated by teachers and believed that something more complex—perhaps 10 factors—would be necessary to organize the thousands of attributes available in the natural language. I asked Norman whether he had considered that a more complex solution might emerge, had he cast his net more widely, rather than limiting his study to only 20 scales. Interestingly, he agreed and subsequently extended his investigations, beginning with an expansion of the original list of personality terms of Allport and Odbert to 2,800 trait-descriptive terms (Norman, 1967), convinced, as others have been, that there simply must be factors beyond the five found in his early studies. Subsequently, Goldberg (1990) examined this generally held conviction and found that it simply did not square with reality; various analyses of 75 trait scales based on 1,431 items demonstrated remarkable robustness for five-factor solutions but not for more complex solutions.

In two studies very similar in procedure to the earlier studies of Cattell (1947, 1948), Borgatta (1964) collected ratings of sorority and fraternity members, using rating scales based on the five-factor solutions of Tupes and Christal. However, unlike those investigators, who had used Cattell's complex bipolar scales, Borgatta designed his own rating scales, which consisted of brief sentence stems (e.g., "Is assertive"). Analysis of 34 such scales produced five clear factors, to which Borgatta gave the names Assertiveness, Likeability, Responsibility, Emotionality, and Intelligence.

Soon thereafter, Smith (1967) employed 42 bipolar rating scales based on the work of Allport and Odbert (1936) and Cattell (1947, 1948), the subjects being college first-year students who were rated by other members of their study group. Factor analysis of the correlations of three independent groups of students revealed a very stable structure. Smith interpreted the factors as Extraversion, Agreeableness, Emotionality, Strength of Character—which would be labeled Conscientiousness today—and Refinement, which can be interpreted as an aspect of Intellect/Openness.

The Nonconformist: Hans Eysenck

Beginning with his analyses of neurotic World War II soldiers, Eysenck (1947) has held steadily to a model of personality that stands in sharp contrast to his contemporaries, Cattell, Thurstone, and Guilford. However complex personality eventually might prove to be, Eysenck proposed to begin with two broad dimensions, Extraversion and Neuroticism. Subsequently, a third dimension, Psychoticism, was added (Eysenck, 1955). Eysenck has held that these three "super factors" exist at a rather high level of abstraction, organizing traits, such as rigidity and accuracy, which are more specific. From the beginning, Eysenck (1960) has distinguished between intelligence and the nonintellective aspects of individual differences, or *temperament*: "There is the case of intelligence . . . which is more or less orthogonal to all the dimensions so far discussed" (p. 115).

The Eysenck model has four dimensions in all, then, if we include, rather than set aside, the domain of Intellect, and compared with the analyses of Thurstone, Cattell, and Guilford, very parsimonious—and very close to the five-factor model (Digman, 1990). The principal difference between the Eysenck model and the five-factor model—other than the setting aside of Intellect—is the fusion of Agreeableness and Conscientiousness into the single dimension of (Freedom from) Psychoticism. As Eysenck (1992) has pointed out, *scales* that are constructed of items that denote these two factors are often rather well correlated (Costa, McCrae, & Dye, 1991). The question remains whether we shall regard these as sufficiently distinct to warrant separate identities. I believe that the evidence (Costa & McCrae, 1992; Digman, 1990; Goldberg, 1990) is very much in favor of the Big Five distinction between these two factors.

The Era of Skepticism

The 1960s ushered in a widespread reaction to traditional personality assessment that in many ways was destructive. Thus, it is not surprising that Norman's work was often dismissed. The influential book by Mischel (1968), *Personality and Assessment,* was not only critical of the trait approach, but also it offered an explanation of the five factors obtained by Norman and by Tupes and Christal in terms of superficial "stereotypes" held by viewers of others, stereotypes that had little to do with actual behavior. Even more destructive were the radical behaviorists of that time, who with the born-again zeal of John Watson would dismiss not only traits but also all mental phenomena from the purview of a scientific psychology, which should confine itself to the objective task of simply counting responses to stimuli. Often citing (misleadingly) the character studies of Hartshorne and May (1928), the detractors coined the term "personality coefficient," for the typical validity coefficient of .30 or less, found in many studies concerned with the predictive validity of personality trait measures. After squaring this value, the explanatory power of personality traits was deemed to be lamentably trivial. Not only were traits mostly figments of observers' imaginations, they had little practical value in the real world of behavior prediction and management.

A Cacophony of Voices

Until recent times, then, the psychometric approach to the essential dimensionality of personality constructs had failed to produce a generally accepted model. One system held that the structure was very complex, with a minimum of 16 essential personality factors. Another offered a structure that was quite simple, a model with only 3 factors. There were also occasional reports of solutions with anywhere between 2 and 10 factors. Small wonder that a review (Cronbach, 1970) of these efforts to bring order to the field of personality traits by way of factor analysis should conclude that this was a long way from serious science; indeed, Cronbach suggested that "game" (p. 523) was the word that best summarized the results of the factor approach to personality.

The Renaissance of the Five-Factor Model

Personality psychology rediscovered the five-factor model in the 1980s. At a convention of the Western Psychological Association in Honolulu in 1980, Lewis Goldberg joined Naomi Takemoto-Chock, Andrew Comrey, and me in a symposium on factor models of personality. Goldberg (1980) had begun to appreciate the essential wisdom of Norman's (1963) "adequate taxonomy," having spent several years, as he subsequently put it (Goldberg, 1993), "wandering as if in a fog" (p. 29) in his attempts to reconcile his five-factor analyses of self- and peer ratings (prompted by earlier work with Norman) with a seductive three-factor analysis espoused by Peabody (1967, 1970). I had spent two decades in trying to make some sense out of teachers' ratings of children, occasionally—on my pessimistic days—thinking that the structure could support no more than seven factors, and finding evidence—on my optimistic days—for a 10-factor model about which I can now see that I was much too fond, mostly because it was *my* model. At this symposium, we both announced our somewhat reluctant conclusions: Five-factor solutions were remarkably stable across studies, whereas more complex solutions were not.

Shaking the dust from his Hawaiian sandals, Goldberg (1983) carried the "new" message across the continent to a research seminar organized by Paul Costa at the Gerontology Research Center in Baltimore. Paul Costa and Robert McCrae, who had developed a three-factor view of personality (Costa & McCrae, 1976) in terms of three clusters (Neuroticism, Extraversion, Openness), were quickly persuaded to add Agreeableness and Conscientiousness, and the first inventory based on the Big Five factors was launched (Costa & McCrae, 1985).

Soon thereafter, many other researchers were also persuaded of the essential usefulness of this Big Five model. Whereas the original work by Fiske, Tupes and Christal, Norman, Borgatta, and Smith had been almost completely overlooked by personality researchers and theorists, the energetic efforts of research and publication by Costa and McCrae made it certain that the model would this time around be seriously examined. In rather short order, this energetic pair (Costa, 1991; Costa & McCrae, 1985, 1988a, 1988b, 1992; Costa, McCrae, & Dye, 1991; McCrae, 1992; McCrae & Costa, 1985; McCrae & John, 1992) produced studies that offered convincing evidence of the presence of some or all of the Big Five in many well-known inventories, such as the Personality Research Form (Jackson, 1984), the California Q-Set (Block, 1961), and the Myers–Briggs Type Indicator (Myers & McCauley, 1985).

Quick to adopt the model, to cite but a few authors, were John (1989, 1990), Angleitner and Ostendorf (1994), Borkenau and Ostendorf (1989, 1990), and Wiggins and Pincus (1993). During the same time, Goldberg's (1990, 1992, 1993) continuing studies of the language of personality, and a focus chapter on the model in the *Annual Review of Psychology* (Digman, 1990) helped to bring the model to the attention of a wide audience.

The History of the Model:
Curious? Yes. Unusual? No.

At the beginning of this chapter, I suggested that the history of this model, with its occasional discovery here and there, its long struggle with contending views, and its rediscovery a generation after its initial appearance, is "curious," seemingly implying that its slow acceptance is unusual in science. Quite the contrary. Ways of thinking about a scientific field—I shall call them *intellectual perspectives*—change glacially. Witness the history of the notion of plate tectonics in geophysics; acceptance came long after the death of Wegener, who proposed the model in the 1920s to fellow geophysicists, who were not only skeptical but also openly derisive. Or consider the long resistance to Darwin's theory of evolution by natural selection on the part of prominent biologists of the 19th century. In medicine Semmelweis, an Austrian physician, concluded that childbed fever, which sometimes reached epidemic proportions in maternity hospitals in the early 19th century, could be avoided by the simple expedient of washing one's hands. The notion was regarded as absurd by his fellow physicians. And in music, another creative field, Brahms reported the audience reaction to his Piano Concerto Number No. 1 as disapproving silence, "broken by the sound of a few hands clapping." Perhaps the most famous disapproval of a new form of music occurred in 1912, when a Parisian audience greeted Stravinsky's *Rite of Spring* with a near riot.

It seems, then, that any new intellectual perspective, whether in science or in the arts, will often be greeted at first with skepticism, if not downright hostility. And perhaps one generation, with its accustomed intellectual set of mind, must pass and a new generation come on the scene for new perspectives to be seriously considered.

There is also the *personal* aspect of science. Supposedly, science is *impersonal*. Yet, as Allport (1961) might have put it, in his concept of "extension of the self," recognition for the scientist comes when his or her name becomes attached to some finding or theory. It is not "the theory of evolution by natural selection" but *Darwin's* theory, *Einstein's* theory of relativity, and *Freud's* theory of the unconscious. And in the concert hall, one does not listen to "a concerto written by a composer of the last century, one Ludwig van Beethoven"; it is *Beethoven's* Concerto No. 3. In science, in art, and in music, these works of ours can become as essential to our conceptions of self as are our own family members, and a suggestion that a model with which we have been identified could profit from correction or that it is basically flawed can marshal a full range of defenses.

Finally, one may note that the instruments employed in any scientific field improve as the years pass: Turn-of-the-century physicists could never have found evidence for the neutrino, given the instruments available in the first two decades of the century, nor could Webb have used a computer to analyze his correlations by way of principal-axis factor analysis with varimax rotation. By contrast, Goldberg (1990), working with a set of 75 self-report variables, based on 187 subjects, checked on the occasionally voiced criticism that the results of factor studies depend on the particulars of the analysis (common factor analysis vs. principal components, orthogonal vs. oblique rotation) by analyzing the correlations in several ways, including the number of factors. Before the advent of computers, a study of this magnitude was simply out of the question. Another example is parallel analysis, an excellent procedure for estimating the number of components or factors to retain, demands the creation and analysis of several sets of random variables. Certainly, we cannot fault earlier investigators for not using instruments and techniques available to us today, any more than we would fault Galileo for failing to observe Neptune with his primitive telescope.

Nonetheless, several investigators were tantalizingly close to the Big Five by the end of the 1930s. How did it happen that we were thrown off the track for a generation? In retrospect, one may discern two pervasive influences, both of which were related to factor-analysis methodology.

One has already been noted—Thurstone's mistaken assumption that factor overextraction was a sound principle. Unfortunately, it was not, nor was the "eigenvalue of one" principle, which often leads to overextraction (Zwick & Velicer, 1986). Although one may very meaningfully hold the view that the causes of any bit of behavior are many and very complexly related to behavior, the corollary that one may find many of these causes by factor analysis can easily lead the unwary astray. Closely related is traditional hypothesis testing; with a sufficient number of observations, almost any null hypothesis may be rejected (Kaiser, 1974). The essential question is not whether some experimental effect or interesting factor is significant; the basic question is, Will these results replicate? There is only one way to answer this important question, and that, of course, is to do the replication—at a minimum of two independent studies. Even better would be several studies by different investigators, whose results may then be compared and a consensus drawn via meta-analysis (Schmidt, 1992).

A second influence is related to the first. Whereas the slow, cautious approach that characterized early studies, such as Cattell's (1933) study of temperament and Eysenck's (1947) early work, was initially dictated by the lack of computers, the availability of high-speed computational equipment from the late 1950s on made possible these overly complex studies, such as (*mea culpa*) my own first attempts (Digman, 1963) at factoring teachers' ratings of schoolchildren. Typically, these overly complex solutions did not replicate, and mine were no exception.

However, the past decade indicates that we are back on course. With the Big Five, we have a model that has shown robustness across cultures (e.g., Church & Katibak, 1989), across media (e.g., Costa & McCrae, 1988b), across age groups (e.g., Digman & Takemoto-Chock, 1981), and which offers a model for unifying the field of personality attributes (Goldberg, 1993). Last, but hardly least important, the model has suggested its use in fields as diverse as evolutionary psychology (Buss, 1991), clinical psychology (Costa & Widiger, 1994), and personnel selection (Barrick & Mount, 1991).

This is not a complete theory of personality—nor does it claim to be. Much remains to be done. For example, do these broad dimensions of personality emerge out of temperament differences at an early age? How are they modified by early experience? To what degree can conscientiousness, for instance, be increased by special training? Does this model suggest a need for new theories of personality development and functioning, or do classical theories, such as ego psychology and social learning theory, suffice to explain individual differences in these five dimensions?

We have at last a meaningful and robust model for personality attributes. The perspectives presented in this volume provide theoretical contexts in which these and other questions may be meaningfully explored within a common model. We may now look forward to the fruits such studies may bear.

Notes

1. Strictly speaking, a distinction may be made between the Big Five model based on word meanings (the lexical hypothesis of Goldberg, 1993) and the model espoused by Costa and McCrae (1992) based on self-report of behaviors.

2. A copy of this analysis may be obtained from the author.

References

Allport, G. W. (1961). *Pattern and growth in personality.* New York: Holt, Rinehart & Winston.

Allport, G. W., & Odbert, H. S. (1936). Trait names: A psycho-lexical study. *Psychological Monographs, 47*(1, Whole No. 211).

Angleitner, A., & Ostendorf, F. (1994). Temperament and the big five factors of personality. in C. F. Halverson, Jr., G. A. Kohnstamm, & R. P. Martin (Eds.), *The developing structure of temperament and personality from infancy to adulthood* (pp. 69–90). Hillsdale, NJ: Erlbaum.

Barrick, M. R., & Mount, M. K. (1991). The Big Five personality dimensions and job performance: A meta-analysis. *Personnel Psychology, 44,* 1–26.

Block, J. (1961). *The Q-sort methodology in personality assessment.* Springfield, IL: Thomas.

Borgatta, E. F. (1964). The structure of personality characteristics. *Behavioral Science, 9,* 8–17.

Borkenau, P., & Ostendorf, F. (1989). Untersuchungen zum Fünf-Factoren-Modell der Persönlichkeit und seiner diagnostoschen Erfassung [Investigations of the five-factor model of personality and its assessment]. *Zeitschrift für Diferentielle und Diagnostische Psychologie, 10,* 239–251.

Borkenau, P., & Ostendorf, F. (1990). Comparing exploratory and confirmatory factor analysis: A study on the 5-factor model of personality. *Personality and Individual Differences, 11,* 515–524.

Buss, D. M. (1991). Evolutionary psychology. In M. R. Rosenzweig & L. W. Porter (Eds.), *Annual review of psychology* (Vol. 42, pp. 459–491). Palo Alto, CA: Annual Reviews.

Cattell, R. B. (1933). Temperament tests. II: Tests. *British Journal of Psychology, 23,* 308–329.

Cattell, R. B. (1944). Interpretation of the twelve primary personality factors. *Character and Personality, 13,* 55–91.

Cattell, R. B. (1947). Confirmation and clarification of the primary personality factors. *Psychometrika, 12,* 197–220.

Cattell, R. B. (1948). The primary personality factors in women compared with those in men. *British Journal of Psychology, 1,* 114–130.

Cattell, R. B. (1950). *Personality: A systematic theoretical and factual study.* New York: McGraw-Hill.

Cattell, R. B. (1957). *Personality and motivation structure and measurement.* Yonkers, NY: World Book.

Church, A. T., & Katibak, M. S. (1989). Internal, external, and self-report structure of personality in a non-Western culture: An investigation of cross-language and cross-cultural generalizability. *Journal of Personality and Social Psychology, 57,* 857–872.

Costa, P. T., Jr. (1991). Clinical use of the Five-Factor Model: An introduction. *Journal of Personality Assessment, 57,* 393–398.

Costa, P. T., Jr., & McCrae, R. R. (1976). Age differences in personality structure: A cluster analysis approach. *Journal of Gerontology, 31,* 564–570.

Costa, P. T., Jr., & McCrae, R. R. (1985). *The NEO Personality Inventory manual.* Odessa, FL: Psychological Assessment Resources.

Costa, P. T., Jr., & McCrae, R. R. (1988a). From catalog to classification: Murray's needs and the five-factor model. *Journal of Personality and Social Psychology, 55,* 258–265.

Costa, P. T., Jr., & McCrae, R. R. (1988b). Personality in adulthood: A six-year longitudinal study of self-reports and spouse ratings on the NEO Personality Inventory. *Journal of Personality and Social Psychology, 54,* 853–863.

Costa, P. T., Jr., & McCrae, R. R. (1992). Four ways five factors are basic. *Personality and Individual Differences, 13,* 653–665.

Costa, P. T., Jr., McCrae, R. R., & Dye, D. A. (1991). Facet scales for Agreeableness and Conscientiousness: A revision of the NEO Personality Inventory. *Personality and Individual Differences, 12,* 887–898.

Costa, P. T., Jr., & Widiger, T. A. (Eds.). (1994). *Personality disorders and the Five-Factor Model of personality.* Washington, DC: American Psychological Association.

Cronbach, L. J. (1970). *Essentials of psychological testing* (3rd ed.). New York: Harper & Row.

Digman, J. M. (1963). Principal dimensions of child personality as inferred from teachers' judgments. *Child Development, 34,* 43–60.

Digman, J. M. (1990). Personality structure: The emergence of the Five-Factor Model. In M. R. Rosenzweig & L. W. Porter (Eds.), *Annual review of psychology* (Vol. 41, pp. 417–440). Palo Alto, CA: Annual Reviews.

Digman, J. M., & Takemoto-Chock, N. K. (1981). Factors in the natural language of personality: Reanalysis, comparison, and interpretation of six major studies. *Multivariate Behavioral Research, 16,* 149–160.

Eysenck, H. J. (1947). *Dimensions of personality.* London: Routledge & Kegan Paul.

Eysenck, H. J. (1955). Psychiatric diagnosis as a psychological and statistical problem. *Psychological Reports, 1,* 3–17.

Eysenck, H. J. (1960). *The structure of human personality.* London: Methuen.

Eysenck, H. J. (1992). Four ways five factors are *not* basic. *Personality and Individual Differences, 13,* 667–673.

Fiske, D. W. (1949). Consistency of the factorial structure of personality ratings from different sources. *Journal of Abnormal and Social Psychology, 44,* 329–344.

Garnett, J. C. M. (1919). General ability, cleverness, and purpose. *British Journal of Psychology, 9,* 345–366.

Goldberg, L. R. (1980, May). *Some ruminations about the structure of individual differences: Developing a common lexicon for the major characteristics of human personality.* Symposium presentation at the meeting of the Western Psychological Association, Honolulu, HI.

Goldberg, L. R. (1983, June). *The magical number five, plus or minus two: Some considerations on the dimensionality of personality descriptors.* Paper presented at a research seminar, Gerontology Research Center, NIA/NIH, Baltimore, MD.

Goldberg, L. R. (1990). An alternative "Description of personality": The Big-Five factor structure. *Journal of Personality and Social Psychology, 59,* 1216–1229.

Goldberg, L. R. (1992). The development of markers of the Big-Five factor structure. *Psychological Assessment, 4,* 26–42.

Goldberg, L. R. (1993). The structure of phenotypic personality traits. *American Psychologist, 48,* 26–34.

Goldberg, L. R., & Digman, J. M. (1994). Revealing structure in the data: Principles of exploratory factor analysis. In S. Strack & M. Lorr (Eds.), *Differentiating abnormal and normal personality* (pp. 216–242). New York: Springer.

Guilford, J. P., & Guilford, R. B. (1936). Personality factors S, E, and M, and their measurement. *Journal of Personality, 34,* 21–36.

Guilford, J. P., & Guilford, R. B. (1939a). Personality factors D, R, T, and A. *Journal of Abnormal and Social Psychology, 34,* 21–36.

Guilford, J. P., & Guilford, R. B. (1939b). Personality factors N and GD. *Journal of Abnormal and Social Psychology, 34,* 239–248.

Hartshorne, H., & May, M. A. (1928). *Studies in deceit.* New York: Macmillan.

Jackson, D. N. (1984). *Personality Research Form manual.* Port Huron, MI: Research Psychologists Press.

John, O. P. (1989). Towards a taxonomy of personality descriptors. In D. M. Buss & N. Cantor (Eds.), *Personality psychology: Recent trends and emerging directions* (pp. 261–271). New York: Springer-Verlag.

John, O. P. (1990). The "Big Five" factor taxonomy: Dimensions of personality in the natural language and in questionnaires. In L. A. Pervin (Ed.), *Handbook of personality: Theory and research* (pp. 66– 100). New York: Guilford Press.

Kaiser, H. F. (1974). A review of Lawley, D. N., & Maxwell, A. E. Factor analysis as a statistical method. *Educational and Psychological Measurement, 36,* 586–589.

Lovell, C. (1945). A study of the factor structure of thirteen personality variables. *Educational and Psychological Measurement, 5,* 335–350.

McCrae, R. R. (1992). Editor's introduction to Tupes and Christal. *Journal of Personality, 60,* 217–219.

McCrae, R. R., & Costa, R. R. (1985). Updating Norman's "adequate taxonomy": Intelligence and personality dimensions in natural language and in questionnaires. *Journal of Personality and Social Psychology, 49,* 710–721.

McCrae, R. R., & John, O. P. (1992). An introduction to the five-factor model and its applications. *Journal of Personality, 60,* 175–215.

Mischel, W. (1968). *Personality and assessment.* New York: Wiley.

Myers, I. B., & McCauley, M. H. (1985). *Manual: A guide to the development and use of the Myers–Briggs Type Indicator.* Palo Alto, CA: Consulting Psychologists Press.

Norman, W. T. (1963a, October). *Replicated personality factors in peer ratings.* Paper presented at the meeting of the Society of Multivariate Experimental Psychology, Boulder, CO.

Norman, W. T. (1963b). Toward an adequate taxonomy of personality attributes: Replicated factor structure in peer nomination personality ratings. *Journal of Abnormal and Social Psychology, 66,* 574–583.

Norman, W. T. (1967). *2800 personality trait descriptors: Normative operating characteristics for a university population.* Ann Arbor, MI: University of Michigan, Department of Psychology.

Peabody, D. (1967). Trait inferences: Evaluative and descriptive aspects. *Journal of Personality and Social Psychology Monographs, 7*(Whole No. 644).

Peabody, D. (1970). Evaluative and descriptive aspects in personality perception: A reappraisal. *Journal of Personality and Social Psychology, 46,* 639–646.

Schmidt, F. L. (1992). What do data really mean? *American Psychologist, 46,* 1173–1181.

Smith, G. M. (1967). Usefulness of peer ratings of personality in educational research. *Educational and Psychological Measurement, 27,* 967–984.

Spearman, C. (1904). General intelligence, objectively determined and measured. *American Journal of Psychology, 15,* 201–293.

Thurstone, L. L. (1934). The vectors of mind. *Psychological Review, 41,* 1–32.

Thurstone, L. L. (1947). *Multiple factor analysis.* Chicago: University of Chicago Press.

Thurstone, L. L. (1951). The dimensions of temperament. *Psychometrika, 16,* 11–20.

Tupes, E. C., & Christal, R. E. (1961). *Recurrent personality factors based on trait ratings* (USAF ASD Tech. Rep. No. 61–97). Lackland Air Force Base, TX: U.S. Air Force.

Tupes, E. C., & Christal, R. E. (1992). Recurrent personality factors based on trait ratings. *Journal of Personality, 60,* 225–261.

Tupes, E. C., & Kaplan, M. N. (1961). *Similarity of factors underlying peer ratings of socially acceptable, socially unacceptable, and bipolar personality traits* (USAF ASD Tech. Rep. No. 61–48). Lackland Air Force Base, TX: U.S. Air Force.

Webb, E. (1915). Character and intelligence. *British Journal of Psychology Monographs, 1*(3), 1–99.

Wiggins, J. S. (1973). *Personality and prediction: Principles of personality assessment.* Reading, MA: Addison-Wesley.

Wiggins, J. S., & Pincus, A. L. (1993). Personality: Structure and assessment. In M. R. Rosenzweig & L. W. Porter (Eds.), *Annual review of psychology* (Vol. 43, pp. 473–504). Palo Alto, CA: Annual Reviews.

Zwick, W. R., & Velicer, W. F. (1986). Comparison of five rules for determining the number of components to retain. *Psychological Bulletin, 99,* 432–442.

CHAPTER TWO

The Language of Personality: Lexical Perspectives on the Five-Factor Model

GERARD SAUCIER
LEWIS R. GOLDBERG

In the beginning was the Word. . . .
—THE GOSPEL ACCORDING
TO SAINT JOHN

The good Saint did not go back far enough, of course: Before the first word, there had to be something to say. Nonetheless, John's emphasis on semantics foreshadowed some important scientific developments during the 20th century, including the topic of the present chapter—the lexical approach to the representation of phenotypic personality attributes.

Just as humans seem to differ in a nearly infinite number of attributes, personality researchers differ in the *particular* attributes that they find most interesting to study. When questioned about these preferences, many investigators invoke the vague, magical terms "theory" or "theoretical" as their justification, which may mean no more than that someone else has also been interested in the same attribute. For example, why is the attribute called "Openness to Experience" (McCrae & Costa, in press) any more "theoretical" than the attribute "UI(T) 31: Wary Realism" (Cattell, 1957)? What makes the popular twin attributes "Agency" and "Communion" (Bakan, 1966; Wiggins, 1991) more "theoretical" than the attributes "Neuroticism" and "Psychoticism" (Eysenck, 1991)? Indeed, what is there about the attributes "Ego Resiliency" and "Ego Control" (Block & Block, 1980) that makes them more "theoretical" than "Factor I" and "Factor II" in the Big Five factor structure? If the present authors were in charge of the world, we would ban the use of the term "theoretical" (except perhaps in the title of this volume), in favor of more exact terms such as "premises," "assumptions," and "hypotheses," as well as more meaningful distinctions such as "broad versus narrow" and "phenotypic versus genotypic" attributes. We will make use of these distinctions later in this chapter.

The Lexical Hypothesis

In any large realm, one needs a map, lest one wander in circles forever. Because the realm of human attributes is so immense, a map is all the more crucial. In his *Nicomachean Ethics,* Aristotle attempted to provide such a map for human "character" traits, and since his time, others have tried similar mappings. Until the 20th century, however, none of these psychocartographic attempts met with much success. In hindsight, it is apparent that at least two scientific problems had to be solved first, so as to yield (1) a procedure for *sampling* human attributes and (2) a method for *structuring* that sample of attributes. The 20th century provided some tools for solving both problems, with the formulation of the "lexical hypothesis" and the development of the set of statistical techniques generically referred to as "factor analysis."

Over the years, a number of philosophers and linguists have remarked about the "wisdom" embedded in natural languages. For example, the philosopher J. L. Austin (1957) noted that

> our common stock of words embodies all the distinctions men have found worth drawing, and the connexions they have found worth marking, in the lifetimes of many generations: these surely are likely to be more numerous, more sound, since they have stood up to the long test of the survival of the fittest, and more subtle, at least in all ordinary and reasonably practical matters, than any that you or I are likely to think up in our arm-chairs of an afternoon—the most favored alternative method. (p. 8)

Included within "our common stock of words" are a substantial subset of terms that refer to individual differences. In the late 1920s and early 1930s, psychologists began to turn to this repository of personality wisdom as a source of the most important phenotypic human attributes (e.g., Klages, 1926; Allport & Odbert, 1936).

The rationale for this lexical hypothesis was well stated by Cattell (1943):

> The position we shall adopt is a very direct one . . . making only the one assumption that all aspects of human personality which are or have been of importance, interest, or utility have already become recorded in the substance of language. For, throughout history, the most fascinating subject of general discourse, and also that in which it has been most vitally necessary to have adequate, representative symbols, has been human behavior. (p. 483)

Cattell (1957) argued: "Over the centuries, by the pressure of urgent necessity, every aspect of one human being's behavior that is likely to affect another has come to be handled by some verbal symbol—at least in any developed modern language. Although some new words for traits constantly appear, a debris of equivalent but obsolete words constantly falls from the language" (p. 71).

Perhaps the most widely quoted explications of the lexical hypothesis are those of Norman (1963):

> Attempts to construct taxonomies of personality characteristics have ordinarily taken as an initial data base some set of perceptible variations in performance and appearance between persons or within individuals over time and varying situations. By far the most general efforts to specify the domain of phenomena on which to base such a system have proceeded from an examination of the natural language. (p. 574)

Norman (1967) argued that a truly comprehensive (or in his words, "exhaustive") taxonomy of personality attributes must take as its fundamental database

> the set of all perceptible variations in performance and appearance between persons or within individuals over time and varying situations that are *of sufficient social significance, of sufficiently widespread occurrence, and of sufficient distinctiveness to have been encoded and retained as a subset of descriptive predicates in the natural language during the course of its development, growth, and refinement.* (p. 2, italics added)

Some recent critics (e.g., Block, 1995) argue for ignoring this natural repository, because it is used by "novices" (i.e., laypersons) in personality description. We take a different view. "Common speech" may be an imperfect "guide to psychological subtleties" (Allport, 1961, p. 356), but it is a powerful guide to salient phenomena that scientists should not ignore. To discard all lay conceptions, besides being unrealistic, "would require us needlessly to separate ourselves from the vast sources of knowledge gained in the course of human history" (Kelley, 1992, p. 22).

Indeed, scientific concepts often evolve from folk concepts (Sternberg, Conway, Ketron, & Bernstein, 1981; Tellegen, 1993). Even as folk concepts such as height, weight, volume, and age provide basic but not exhaustive (necessary but not sufficient) components for a science of physical differences, likewise personality concepts in the natural language provide basic but not exhaustive (necessary but not sufficient) components for a science of personality attributes.

Recent criticisms of the lexical hypothesis (e.g., Block, 1995; McCrae, 1990; Stagner, 1994) reflect an inadequate understanding of the lexical approach. In this chapter, we will try to provide a clarifying perspective. First we will articulate a set of premises that constitute the essence of the lexical perspective; we will try to demonstrate that these premises are in harmony with major criteria for "good science," such as comprehensiveness, parsimony, testability, and evidence of empirical validation. Although we welcome attempts to refute these premises, we believe they are so well grounded as to be difficult to refute. On the other hand, we shall suggest that the lexical perspective has a finite scope, and is not intended to provide a complete or exhaustive "theory of personality."

Along the way, we shall suggest a few refinements of terminology appropriate to the lexical perspective. We turn first to a crucial distinction imported into psychology from biology.

1. *Personality language refers to phenotypes and not genotypes.* The concept of *genotype* refers to underlying (causal) properties, whereas the concept of *phenotype* refers to observable (surface) characteristics. As a rule, observers of personality are not equipped with those devices necessary to observe genotypes. Thus, our perceived personality attributes are phenotypic. Several subtle but important distinctions follow.

First, the language of personality provides a framework for

description, but not necessarily for explanation. A genotype provides an explanation for a phenotype, but a particular phenotype has no necessary implication for a particular genotype; there need be no one-to-one correspondence between phenotypic and genotypic patterns. Phenotypic attributes of personality may be accounted for by genotypic constructs related to nature (e.g., our genetic inheritance), to nurture (e.g., experience, conditioning, social learning, culture), or more likely some combination of genetic and environmental influences. The lexical perspective leads to data that need explaining, not necessarily to the modes of explanation. It "makes no explicit assumptions (or claims) about the ontological status of traits or about the causal origins of the regularities to which they refer" (John & Robins, 1994, p. 138). Because it describes without venturing to explain, the lexical perspective, compared to some other approaches in the study of personality, may be less prone to encourage the "fundamental attribution error" (Ross, 1977) of an irrational preference for dispositional over situational explanations of behavior.

Second, the lexical perspective is not an instance of "trait theory" (Pervin, 1994), although "trait theorists" (if there be such creatures) might profit from attention to the lexical perspective. "Trait theory," a rubric that may have no meaning outside introductory personality texts (Goldberg, 1994), is held to assume that personality characteristics are relatively stable over time and across situations. The lexical perspective itself does not require these assumptions, having no staked-out position on whether the phenotypic attributes encoded in language are verifiably stable.

Third, those phenotypic personality characteristics upon which the lexical perspective focuses are really better described as "attributes" than as "traits." Like an awkward tourist in an unfamiliar land, the word "trait" carries too much baggage into studies of phenotypic personality language. "Trait" is a term used to describe genotypes as well as phenotypes (e.g., "sickle-cell trait"), and was used by Allport (1937) to denote a "bona fide mental structure" that explained behavior (p. 289). Moreover, calling a characteristic a "trait" already implies that the characteristic is stable, which is a matter for empirical verification, rather than a priori presumption. A model of attributes should not be equated with a model of traits (Goldberg, 1993a). The use of "attribute" makes a clearer reference to phenotype, without any implications about the stability of that phenotype, and without unnecessary implications as to genotype.

2. *Phenotypic attributes are encoded in the natural language.* This proposition is the first part of the lexical hypothesis. The phenotypic attributes worth noticing become encoded in language as a word for the attribute appears and is maintained by frequent use. In this respect, language comes to reflect our knowledge of the world, and indeed, language is the prime medium through which we come to "know" personality.

Of course, we need not presume simplistically that this encoding is literal and exact, with exactly one word for one attribute or vice versa, because neither attributes nor words can be assumed to have a discrete, nongraded structure. The meaning of a new word must be defined relative to the rest of the semantic field, and it is likely to include not only synonymy and contrast, but also uniqueness. We can ask of a new word: What new facet of description does it add; to apply a psychometric simile, what is its "discriminant validity"?

As a result of the inevitable interrelations between our language and our understanding of personality, the concepts in everyday use to categorize human actions and practices form a substantial part of the subject matter of personality psychology. The scientific study of personality, even if it reveals errors in lay use of these concepts, will always have to relate back to such folk concepts (Hampson, 1994).

3. *The degree of representation of an attribute in language has some correspondence with the general importance of the attribute.* This proposition is the second part of the lexical hypothesis, and it can be stated in two forms. First is an across-language form: "The more important is an individual difference in human transactions, the more languages will have a term for it" (Goldberg, 1981, p. 142). Second is a within-language form: The more important is such an attribute, the more synonyms and subtly distinctive facets of the attribute will be found *within any one language,* a conjecture proposed by the linguist Zipf (1949). As implied by either form, the lexical perspective entails an indigenous or "emic" research strategy; analyses are carried out separately within each language, without the importation of translated or "etic" selections of variables from some other language.

Thus, the most important phenotypic personality attributes should have a corresponding term in virtually every language. Moreover, in those languages with a rich personality vocabulary, such an attribute will be referenced by some discernible "associative constellation" (Saussure, 1983; p. 174), a dense cluster of loosely synonymous terms. When used in ratings of oneself or others, these terms will be highly intercorrelated and therefore, along with their antonyms, they will tend to define a semantic "factor." Of course, these synonym clusters are not simply redundant reexpressions for the same attribute, but rather bundles of related concepts likely to have a family-resemblance structure (Rosch & Mervis, 1975; Wittgenstein, 1953).

In short, we assume a correspondence between lexical representation and substantive importance. This premise is in keeping with the common assumption among linguists that reference stems from word–object contiguities in experience. Because we typically learn the meaning of a new word by matching it to some object in our experience to which it is applied, those words in frequent use tend to be those frequently judged as applicable to real-life objects (e.g., persons). Although trivial or illusory attributes might become encoded in language, they are less likely to prove useful across associations with many objects (e.g., persons).

However, the correspondence between lexical representation and substantive importance should not be magnified into a "naive realism," in which mental experiences (including words for attributes) are assumed to map precisely the real features of personality and, therefore, because there is a word for an attribute, it must be a real and important one. Nor should this correspondence be diminished by invoking a strong form of linguistic relativity (Whorf, 1956), in which language is assumed to determine perception and, therefore, personality is assumed to exist only in language.

Rather, we propose a moderate "realism." Because the relation between the lexicon and the real world is mediated by those concepts that are expressed as words, and by any potential distorting effects of their perception, the relation is indirect. Lexical representation is not a pure reflection of objective reality, but in cases in which lexical representation is very prominent (such as a large cluster of related words in a language with a large lexicon, or a frequently used word in a language with a small lexicon) the likelihood of objective, real-world reference is very high.

By this logic, the lexical approach should not be extended beyond the identification of those semantic patterns that are heavily emphasized in language. The significance of one isolated personality adjective in a large-lexicon language such as English is very limited, and the extension of the lexical approach to identifying extremely fine-grained, narrow facets of large factors violates the key premise of the approach. Aggregates of words are more significant than isolated words, and familiar and frequently used words are more significant than unfamiliar and infrequently used words.[1]

Given the premise that lexical representation has some correspondence with substantive importance, another proposition logically follows.

4. *The lexical perspective provides an unusually strong rationale for the selection of variables in personality research.* Biased selection of variables is a ubiquitous threat to the validity of personality research. Even as the language can generate an infinite number of distinct sentences (Chomsky, 1957), a virtually infinite number of sentence-length questionnaire items pertinent to personality can be constructed. With so many potential variables, one does not know when one is using a biased selection. In contrast, there is an essentially finite number of single terms that refer to personality in any language, so better grounds might be established for a relatively nonbiased selection from a large set of personality descriptors. In consequence, with natural-language personality-descriptive terms, one can argue that a selection of variables is actually representative of some larger population of variables (cf. Peabody, 1987); such arguments could prove important in defining the content validity of personality measures.

Of course, the population of variables defined by familiar person-descriptive terms may not be the optimal population of variables for all seasons and situations. For example, the hypothetical population of expert-conceived personality variables will likely be somewhat different (cf. Block, 1995), even if there is considerable overlap. Nonetheless, the population of variables defined by the lexical perspective has the advantage of being little affected by short-term intellectual fads and fashions. Although faddish terms appear and disappear on the surface of the semantic field within decades, the overall framework of language is comparatively conservative and slow-changing, and most personality terms have been used in a recognizably similar way for centuries.[2]

With a relatively unbiased selection of variables, an investigator minimizes prestructuring data that would otherwise produce a facile "confirmation" of prior expectations. As is now well known, research findings depend on the particular set of variables that an investigator chooses to include and exclude. The literature in personality psychology is replete with reports from well-intentioned investigators who have repeatedly "confirmed" their preferred models, using their preferred selection of variables; these investigators are frequently puzzled and frustrated when others, using other selections of variables, remain unconvinced. Bolstered by the trend in human nature toward confirmation of prior expectations, arbitrary variable-selection procedures contribute to the dissonance in personality research. The lexical approach, in contrast, is surely the single approach in personality psychology that best minimizes prestructuring, since the all-important step of variable selection can be taken out of the investigator's hands and delegated instead to dictionaries or aggregated raters (Goldberg & Saucier, 1995). In this respect, the lexical perspective offers one corrective to the encroachment of anchoring effects (Tversky & Kahneman, 1974) and confirmation bias (Einhorn & Hogarth, 1978) into the science of personality.

However, in order to specify a population of lexical variables, one must confront a few difficult issues. First, not all person-descriptive terms would satisfy everyone's criteria for being "personality" relevant. Investigators with narrow definitions of the concept of personality might well choose to exclude physical descriptors (e.g., *tall*), appearance descriptors (e.g., *good-looking*), primarily evaluative terms (e.g., *excellent*), and descriptors of social roles (e.g., *professional*), social effects (e.g., *popular*), or temporary states (e.g., *embarrassed*). Because most of these categories have no clear boundaries separating them from the category of personality attributes (Chaplin, John, & Goldberg, 1988), inclusion and exclusion criteria must be developed to specify the subpopulation of lexical personality variables within the larger population of lexicalized person-descriptors. Investigations are needed to discover the effects of differing variable-inclusion criteria on the resulting lexical findings.

Second, the English language contains many terms whose use in person-description is ambiguous or metaphorical (e.g., *elliptical, snaky, stygian*) and many terms that are obscure and difficult (e.g., *clavering, gnathonic, theromorphic*). It is usually assumed that the meanings of such terms overlap with the set of those that are more commonly used, and therefore they are systematically omitted from most analyses. On the other hand, if one questions this assumption, one might test it by providing dictionary definitions of all terms (Goldberg & Kilkowski, 1985).

Third, person-description employs different parts of speech, including nouns (e.g., "*He's a maverick*"; "*She's a jewel*") and verbs (e.g., "*She often argues*"; "*He never gossips*"), as well as adjectives. Moreover, some languages have few or even no adjectives (Dixon, 1977). On which parts of speech ought we to concentrate?

5. *Person-description and the sedimentation of important differences in language both work primarily through the adjective function.* Dixon (1977) pointed out that, although the word classes noun and verb appear to be universal (cf. Croft, 1991), a number of languages (e.g., Hausa, Telugu) have very few adjectives in general and none referring to human propensities. Moreover, one can find languages (e.g., Yurok) with no adjectives at all. However, Dixon found "adjectival concepts" in all of the languages he surveyed; such terms (1) describe "some important but noncriterial property of an object" and (2) "distinguish between two members of the same species that are described by a single common noun" (p. 63). Similarly, dictionary definitions of "adjective" include its use as (1) a modifier of nouns to denote a quality of the thing named and (2) the designation of a particular thing as distinct from something else. Wierzbicka (1986) has identified the adjective, where such a class does appear, with the denotation of single properties that can be applied to a broad range of entities, in varying degrees or amounts (e.g., *bold, bolder, boldest*). Adjectives attribute qualities or properties, whereas nouns categorize and make reference to objects or events, and verbs identify processes, such as motion, vision, communication, and possession (Miller & Johnson-Laird, 1976).

In some languages (e.g., Dyirbal), this adjective function is carried out entirely through adjectives, whereas in others, the function may be carried out mostly through nouns or verbs. English, like other Indo-European languages, appears to fall between these extremes; it has a very large adjective class, but the adjective function is sometimes carried out through nouns and verbs. When one says "He is a maverick" or "She often argues," one is both (1) describing non-criterial properties of an object (i.e., a person) and (2) distinguishing between members of the same species. Thus, one is carrying out an adjective function through a noun or through a verb. The concept of "adjective function" helps account for differences between nouns that represent a kind of entity combining many features (e.g., *child, woman*) and nouns that serve to identify a single property (e.g., *liar, birdbrain*) and thus function more like adjectives (Wierzbicka, 1986).[3] Evidence cited by Dixon (1977) indicates that, across languages, the adjective function of describing human propensities is more often taken over by nouns, especially abstract attribute nouns (e.g., *skill, generosity*), than by verbs.

Based on such evidence, we propose that adjectives are the prototypical and central repositories of the sedimentation of important individual differences into the natural language. Person-description, as a description of the qualities and characteristics of an object, is inherently an adjective function, although it can be carried out using other word classes. Therefore, the lexical perspective on personality is properly focused on the adjective function. In most languages, this perspective will be adjective-centered, but lexical researchers need to be alert to potential variations: The adjective function of describing kinds of individual differences in certain languages may operate largely through nouns or even verbs.

In most Indo-European languages, and almost certainly in English, personality descriptions found in formal written discourse include far more adjectives than nouns, whereas personality-type nouns are used mostly in informal contexts, especially in spoken conversation. English type nouns tend to be evaluatively more highly polarized than adjectives (e.g., *saint, devil*); unlike adjectives, such nouns most frequently refer to undesirable attributes (e.g., *jerk, bozo*); and many of them are slang expressions that pop into and out of contemporary discourse far more rapidly than adjectives. We assume that the range of attributes incorporated in the total set of personality-type nouns (not to mention personality-attribute nouns) overlaps largely with that of adjectives, a conjecture that we are now subjecting to empirical test.

Personality-relevant verbs present much greater difficulties. The personality implications of most transitive verbs are prohibitively ambiguous, without clarifying the object of the verb (e.g., *enjoys* compared to the far less ambiguous *enjoys life,* or *enjoys loud parties,* or *enjoys violence*). Moreover, some of the most common verbs (e.g., *comes, goes*) are "deictic," or only ambiguously interpretable without "knowledge of the context in which the communication occurs" (Miller & Johnson-Laird, 1976, p. 395). Indeed, Miller and Johnson-Laird attempted an extensive psycholinguistic analysis of English verbs in terms of their implications for understanding human cognition, but they concluded that verbs have complex interrelations, often lying at the intersections of semantic fields. Similarly, other investigators have noted that verbs appear to form associations with members of other word classes more readily than with one another (Deese, 1965), and verbs seem to be organized into much looser associational networks than are adjectives and nouns (Kiss, 1973). As a consequence, we question the usefulness of including most classes of uncontextualized verbs as stimuli for person-descriptions.[4]

6. *The structure of person-descriptions in phrases and sentences is closely related to that based on single words.* One critique sometimes made of the lexical perspective concerns its focus on single, isolated words. For example, McCrae (1990) argued that the allegedly fundamental dimension of Openness to Experience has very few corresponding adjectives in English, a conclusion that was later questioned by Saucier (1992b). If McCrae is correct, and therefore it is necessary to use phrases, sentences, paragraphs, and technical jargon to describe an allegedly fundamental attribute, perhaps there is something wrong with the use of single terms to study the structure of personality attributes.

We acknowledge that finer and subtler thoughts can be expressed in phrases, sentences, and paragraphs (not to mention technical jargon) than in single words. We acknowledge also that personality measurement must avail itself of such nuanced syntactical constructions in order to measure many significant variables reliably. However, in defining the universe of personality-related attributes, single-word descriptors expressing the adjective function have a clear advantage for several reasons. First, the fundamental lexical hypothesis is focused on words, not on sentences. Second, these single-word descriptors comprise an essentially finite domain, offering an unusually powerful rationale for variable selection. Third, the contrast between single adjectives and questionnaire sentences is easily overstated, when, in fact, the syntax of personality-questionnaire items is typically not complex. For example, on the Revised NEO Personality Inventory (NEO-PI-R; Costa & McCrae, 1992), dozens of items are simply person-descriptive adjectives preceded by such phrases as "I am," "I am not," "I sometimes (or often or rarely) feel," and "I am known to be." Indeed, that 240-item inventory includes at least 110 personality adjectives, as well as at least 19 attribute nouns, 4 type nouns, and 3 adverbs constructed from adjectives. Nor is that inventory atypical; many questionnaire items include personality-descriptive adjectives. As a consequence, the deep structure of single terms and of more complex statements may be far more similar than their surface appearances would suggest.

Moreover, research on language suggests that single terms often function holophrastically; that is, they can incorporate complex ideas that are normally expressed in sentences (Macnamara, 1972; Paivio & Begg, 1981). For example, in the telegraphic and holophrastic speech of 2-year-olds, adults can typically infer full-sentence meanings (e.g., "Candy" meaning "I want some candy") and similarly infer meanings from the holophrastic speech of other adults (e.g., "Good" meaning "That is good"). When subjects describe a target using a list of adjectives, their instructions prime them to generate certain implied sentences (e.g., "Courageous" meaning "I am typically courageous"), in effect controlling for conditionals, contextualizations, and specifications.

Indeed, one can best understand the language of personality as a semantic hierarchy consisting of words and phrases at different levels of abstraction versus specification (John, Hampson, & Goldberg, 1991). At the highest level is pure evaluation (*good* vs. *bad*), which can be indexed by some linear composite of Big Five Factors II, III, IV, and V—Factor I being reasonably neutral on the evaluation continuum (Saucier, 1992a, 1994c). At a lower level, but still way up in the stratosphere, are the broad Big Five domains themselves, with the 90 facets of the AB5C model (Hofstee, De Raad, & Goldberg, 1992) located below them. Still quite abstract, but lower in the hierarchy, are all of the single personality descriptors, which in turn can be ordered by their breadth (Hampson, John, & Goldberg, 1986). Each of these single terms (e.g., *extraverted*) can be specified, conditionalized, or contextualized in a host of ways (e.g., *likes to tell jokes at parties*), and it is these myriad specifications that form the basic building blocks of most personality scales and inventories. When viewed in this hierarchical fashion, it is not surprising that analyses of large numbers of diverse personality scales appear to generate much the same factor structure as those based on the higher level single terms.

7. *The science of personality differs from other disciplines in ways that make the lexical perspective particularly germane in this scientific context, yet not in others.* By far the most common criticism of the lexical perspective on personality attributes is of the form: "Imagine how primitive would be the science of physics, chemistry, physiology, or . . . (fill in the blank) if that discipline had restricted its constructs to those found in the natural language." This form of reasoning by analogy might be appropriate if the disciplines being compared were similar in their self-referential nature. However, unlike physics, chemistry, physiology, or . . . (fill in the blank), person judgments are central to the science of personality; our perceptions of ourselves and others form an integral component of the phenomena to be explained by our scientific discipline. Moreover, language serves two functions in this regard: (1) It serves as the only repository of the set of perceptible

individual differences "that are of sufficient social significance, of sufficiently widespread occurrence, and of sufficient distinctiveness" (Norman, 1967, p. 2) to be retained in our collective memory; and (2) language also later serves to constrain our descriptions, if not to some extent our very perceptions, by providing the semantic units necessary for communication to occur.

Said another way, atoms, chemical elements, stars, bodily organs, trees, and other natural objects do not communicate with each other through the medium of language—if they did, you can bet that scientists would want to study their emic, language-based conceptions. Indeed, some of the most fascinating research on animal behavior has focused on communication among primates. However, humans appear to communicate through a uniquely complex language system, a system that acts like a sieve, filtering out concepts that are not of widespread utility, and retaining concepts that are. In the case of personality, those concepts serve to define the core architecture of our discipline. Rarely in the physical and natural sciences can this be said to be true.

The science of personality has as its subject of study socially meaningful behavior patterns; because they are socially meaningful and are interwoven with social action, these patterns are abundantly represented in language. Operational definitions of personality concepts (e.g., *Neuroticism* and *Openness* as scientific constructs) cannot stray far from those definitions collectively represented in the language (e.g., the generally understandable meanings of *neurotic* and *open*), lest they become confusing and useless, and thus inapplicable and ungeneralizable to everyday life.

Although the lexical perspective implies that important individual differences become "socially represented" in language, this social representation in no way implies that these differences are "socially constructed." Again, the lexical perspective suggests that the descriptive classification latent in language partially reflects knowledge of the real extralinguistic world, implying that language has woven into it the world of real human action (cf. Wittgenstein, 1953). Like behavior genetics or ethology, social constructionism is an explanatory approach, whereas the lexical perspective is a purely descriptive one. As Greenwood (1991) points out, "Classificatory descriptions of human actions in terms of social relations and representations are quite *neutral* with respect to explanatory questions" (p. 28). And for all its concern with folk *classifications,* the lexical perspective is in no way committed to folk-psychological causal explanations. The lexical perspective generates a descriptive classification, with no implications as to what conditions enable or influence the characteristics so classified.

8. *The most important dimensions in aggregated personality judgments are the most invariant and universal dimensions—those that replicate across samples of subjects, targets of description, and variations in analytic procedures, as well as across languages.* The lexical perspective can be employed to locate patterns of person perception idiosyncratic to certain types of samples, targets of description, and languages. Of even greater importance, however, the lexical perspective, in line with the scientific goals of comprehensiveness, parsimony, and predictable replication, can be directed toward the discovery of universals. If a personality factor is found only in a certain kind of sample (e.g., men, women, students, children) or in descriptions of a certain kind of target (e.g., self, friend, spouse, child, parent), that attribute would appear less basic than those that replicate across samples and targets. The idiographic pattern is best illuminated by the nomothetic trend.

Moreover, when factor analysis is employed to reduce lexical data to a few parsimonious latent variables, the best solutions are those that are relatively invariant to the procedures used for factor extraction or rotation, at least within the range of reasonably well-accepted methods. A robust and replicable factor solution is one that is so clear and strong that the choice of analytic method becomes unimportant. And because exploratory factor analysis provides a more rigorous replication test than confirmatory analysis, the former technique may often be preferred to the latter. This means that no single analysis is powerful enough to provide evidence of the viability of a factor structure; one needs a number of analyses of at least somewhat different variables in different subject samples. For a more detailed discussion of these principles, see Goldberg and Digman (1994).[5]

Employing the rationale of the lexical perspective, it might be possible to identify a set of universal factors in personality description, that is, relatively invariant factors generated from independent emic studies in many languages (Goldberg, 1981). Of course, the lexical perspective does not necessarily require this hypothesis; it is possible that individual differences are so strongly moderated by culture that no universal lexical dimensions will ever be found.

The hypothesis of universal lexical dimensions includes two separate assumptions. The first concerns the broad dimensionality of the personality attribute space, whereas the second concerns the exact locations of the factor axes within that space. To the extent to which most person descriptors are inherently multidimensional, each a blend of two or more different personality aspects or components, then it is extremely unlikely that factors derived from analyses of different languages will all be found in precisely the same locations, even if the broad dimensionality of the representations turns out to be the same. Rather, one would assume that even small differences between languages in the relative frequencies of terms for particular attributes would inevitably lead to somewhat different factor locations.

One solution to the always somewhat arbitrary problem of factor locations is to accept attribute multidimensionality as a given and to represent the attribute space as a hypersphere, which can be reduced for many purposes to a set of circular structures (e.g., Hofstee et al., 1992). To compare languages, however, it would still be useful to provide some reasonable candidate locations for the reference axes so that different analyses both within and across languages can be sensibly compared. Such special locations can be thought of as orientation guides, such as are provided by the (reasonable yet somewhat arbitrary) polar coordinates by which we circumnavigate the earth.

A considerable body of research has generated a very promising candidate to fill the role of a set of "reasonable locations" for possible universal lexical dimensions—the Big Five factor structure (Goldberg, 1993c). We will now discuss some features of this structure, with the expectation that these features are likely to apply to any set of universal lexical dimensions. To distinguish these generalizations, many of them empirically derived, from the earlier lexical premises, we order them in a separate sequence.

The Big Five Factor Structure

A. *The Big Five personality factors appear to provide a set of highly replicable dimensions that parsimoniously and comprehensively describe most phenotypic individual differences.* To date, research informed by the lexical perspective tends to confirm that personality attributes can be represented at an abstract level, with considerable comprehensiveness and great parsimony, by five broad dimensions. The Big Five have been isolated in relatively similar form in lexical studies of American English (Goldberg, 1990), Dutch (Hofstee & De Raad, 1991), and German (Ostendorf, 1990). Studies are currently under way in languages as diverse as Hungarian, Italian, Czech, Polish, Russian, Tagalog, and Japanese to test the generalization of this five-factor structure to independent personality-related lexicons in non-Germanic languages.

The Big Five model has been distinguished from the five-factor model (FFM) by John and Robins (1993). The Big Five model, which has been derived from lexical data, is a model of personality *attributes* and is therefore descriptive rather than explanatory. Moreover, the Big Five model entails rigorous cross-language replication tests.[6] In contrast, the FFM includes a dispositionalist explanatory hypothesis that the five factors correspond to biological traits ("endogenous basic tendencies"; McCrae & Costa, Chapter 3, this volume). The FFM is based in part on the findings from cluster analyses of the 16 PF (Costa & McCrae, 1976) and in part on two additional dimensions taken directly from the lexically based Big Five model. Research on the FFM has centered on personality questionnaires anchored in English. Although the two models are similar in many respects, they should not be confused.

B. *Given the variety of conceivable exclusion criteria for defining personality attributes, the Big Five are meaningful at all levels, but more comprehensive and parsimonious under narrower definitions of personality.* Allport (1937) has provided a classic discussion of the lack of consensus in defining the meaning of the concept of "personality." Even today, there is still a lack of consensus in what is included as "personality" and what is not. For example, the Dutch lexical team (Brokken, 1978) selected personality terms by means of judgments of their fit into two target sentences: (1) "He or she is . . . by nature" and (2) "He or she is a . . . kind of person." Using the average ratings across both sentence frames, and excluding those terms with average ratings in the lower half of the distribution of all Dutch personality terms, they emerged with an item pool that included primarily terms for stable traits, and that excluded most terms referring to talents and capacities. In contrast, the German lexical team (Angleitner, Ostendorf, & John, 1990), profiting from the experiences of the Dutch, explicitly included terms relating to intellect. The American-English investigators (Norman, 1967; Goldberg, 1982) not only included terms relating to intelligence and other talents, but also included some terms excluded as "attitudes and worldviews" or as "temporary states" by the other two teams. Although none of the three teams included "purely evaluative" and "social effects" terms, Tellegen and Waller (1987) and Waller (in press) have recently argued in favor of including *all* trait, state, attitude, and evaluation terms in lexical analyses. Given that stable traits might be central aspects of the concept of personality, it is clear that there is a graded continuum from terms denoting stable attributes of temperament into those describing temporary states and into those relating to social effects and evaluations, with no clear line of demarcation (Chaplin et al., 1988).

Inasmuch as the Dutch, German, and American teams, despite their differences in exclusion criteria, found a reasonably convergent five-factor structure, it might be provisionally concluded that such differences have relatively few consequences for factor structures. However, such a conclusion would be premature. In our view, the inclusion of large numbers of terms relating to attitudes and worldviews,[7] or terms denoting physical characteristics, could result in additional factors, whereas the inclusion of large numbers of evaluation terms is likely to affect the positions of the rotated factors. Any evaluation term has some (at least small) descriptive reference, so there may be no completely "pure" evaluation terms. A large number of so-called evaluation terms (e.g., *cruel, wicked*) are actually markers of the negative pole of Big Five Factor II (Agreeableness) in ratings of both self and peers (Saucier, 1994a). Many positive evaluation terms may shift semantic reference according to the type of target. For example, the terms *excellent* and *impressive* in self-ratings might signify narcissism, self- esteem, or personal accomplishment, but in ratings of other people, these terms are more likely to signify likability and prosocial attributes (Saucier, 1994b). As long as we accept the usefulness of both types of targets, such evaluation terms will carry with them considerable descriptive ambiguity.

Existing evidence suggests that the Big Five factors will more likely be verified in data sets using narrower rather than broader criteria for the inclusion of attributes. Because "personality" is so hard to define clearly, the broader criteria are not necessarily invalid. Accordingly, the present Big Five structure ought to be considered as an initial approximation (but probably the central hub) of a future model based on a wider array of lexical evidence. Moreover, there is always the yet-untested possibility that some factors beyond the Big Five might be found in analyses of type nouns, attribute nouns, or personality-relevant verbs (cf. De Raad

& Hofstee, 1993; De Raad & Hoskens, 1990; De Raad, Mulder, Kloosterman, & Hofstee, 1988).

In summary, then, the Big Five appears to provide a comprehensive organizing structure for most personality attributes, but the comprehensiveness is not perfect. Clearly, there could be additional dimensions beyond the Big Five. Even in data sets based on adjectives chosen by relatively narrow inclusion criteria, we have isolated a few small outlier dimensions, such as Religiousness, Culture, Prejudice, and Sensuality. These additional dimensions have *far* fewer adjectives defining them, and thus the lexical hypothesis would suggest that they are less important. Nonetheless, we can expect to observe some other outlier dimensions in the future, found either among typical personality adjectives, or in data sets including state or evaluation or social-effect adjectives, or among nouns or verbs performing an adjective function. Some may be unique to a language, population, or type of target. Others might prove to be universal.

C. *The Big Five factors are not necessarily of equal importance and replicability.* The FFM, in many ways parallel to the Big Five model, is often presented as if the five factors were equal in their importance and replicability. But the Big Five model is based on the lexical hypothesis, which provides a rationale for assigning differential importance to one factor or another based on its salience in the natural language. Accordingly, from the lexical perspective, the relative importance of the Big Five factors is an open question.

All of the five factors appear to be remarkably robust by general standards, so it has been relatively easy to proceed as if the five were equal in importance. However, evidence to date suggests that the first three factors (Extraversion, Agreeableness, and Conscientiousness) are typically more easily replicable than the latter two (Emotional Stability and Intellect or Imagination) (Saucier, 1995). And, when one moves from ratings of an evaluatively homogeneous group of targets such as one's close friends to (1) ratings of an evaluatively heterogeneous group of targets, or (2) judgments of the semantic relations among personality attributes, the first three factors become increasingly large relative to the other two (Peabody & Goldberg, 1989). Moreover, as one reduces the number of factors that are rotated to three, one continues to find these first three factors (Goldberg & Rosolack, 1994; Saucier, 1995).

There are a number of reasons for these findings. First of all, there are substantially more English adjectives associated with each of the first three factors than with either of the latter two (Goldberg, 1990). Perhaps, as a consequence, it is easier to find large homogeneous sets of factor markers for the first three factors than for the last two (Goldberg, 1992; Saucier, 1994a). And, the fifth lexical factor (Factor V: Intellect), with the least impressive replication record (cf. Szirmak & De Raad, 1994), appears to be the weakest of the five; initial results from studies of one non-Indo-European language (De Raad & Szirmak, 1994) indicate that it may be necessary to rotate a sixth factor in order to arrive at a clearly represented "Intellect" factor.

McCrae and John (1992) have advocated labeling the five factors by their initials (*E, A, C, N*, and *O*) because of the easy interpretability and high mnemonic value of letters as compared to numbers. This suggestion could lead others to assume that the Big Five are equal in importance and replicability. However, the Roman numerals for the Big Five assigned by Norman (1963) correspond roughly to the order in which they are represented among common English trait terms (cf. Peabody & Goldberg, 1989). It may be no accident that the factor whose replicability is the subject of the greatest controversy is labeled Factor V, the last factor. The retention of the Roman numerals as labels is sensible from the standpoint of the lexical perspective, unless and until evidence indicates no parallel between primacy of numbering and either importance or replicability.

Finally, there is no basis for an arbitrary a priori assumption that the Big Five factors each have the same number of specific "facets." One might suppose that larger and more important factors would include more subordinate facets, but this is still an open question.

D. *The Big Five do not form tight and discrete clusters of variables; rather, as a general rule, each factor represents a major concentration in a continuous distribution of attributes in descriptive space.* As is well known, human perception both of colors and emotions includes not only basic or primary attributes, but also blends of these attributes. Personality description appears to follow suit. For example, Saucier (1992a) and Hofstee et al. (1992) showed that most personality-attribute terms do not relate in a simple manner to only one Big Five factor, but rather correlate substantially with combinations (typically a pair) of factors; that is, personality descriptors are not organized neatly into tight and discrete clusters of variables. Instead, most variables fall in the interstitial areas between the factor poles.

This proclivity to form blends appears to be especially characteristic of Big Five Factors I, II, and IV, moderately characteristic of Factor III, and only weakly characteristic of Factor V, which does not seem to "blend" as easily with the others (Saucier, 1992a); that is, with Factor V one finds fewer variables in the interstitial areas of the two-factor planes (Hofstee et al., 1992); this finding might provide further grounds for regarding the fifth factor in a somewhat different light than the first four.

E. *A complete taxonomy of personality attributes must include both horizontal and vertical features of their meanings.* The horizontal aspect refers to the degree of similarity among attributes at the same hierarchical level (e.g., *humility* involves aspects of both *timidity* and *cooperativeness*). The vertical aspect refers to the hierarchical relations among attributes (e.g., *reliability* is a more abstract and general concept than *punctuality*). It is necessary to think hierarchically about the use of trait measures in applied contexts, but it is equally necessary to think horizontally about basic taxonomic issues (Goldberg, 1993b). Clear hierarchical (vertical) relations between attributes are easy to distinguish for only some of the attributes encoded in the natural language (Hampson et al., 1986; John et al., 1991), whereas horizontal relations are clearly important for a majority of them (cf. Hofstee et al., 1992). The structure of personality attributes is to some degree hierarchical, but to a substantial degree "heterarchical," much like the spectrum of light as it is displayed on a color wheel.

The replication of facets of personality description at a more specific hierarchical level than the Big Five is a daunting task. Between-language differences, the difficulties of translation, and the lack of any clearly agreed-upon methodology for identifying such facets all pose obstacles, but this is an important problem for future research.

F. *Rather than the final chapter for personality research, the Big Five is but an important beginning.* In the face of a growing consensus on the adequacy of the Big Five as an organizing representation for personality attributes, a number of personality researchers of diverse persuasions (e.g., Block, 1995; Paunonen, 1993; Shadel & Cervone, 1993) seem to have reacted defensively to a presumed reduction of all personality research to the Big Five. We hope we can help them breathe a little easier.

The Big Five model does not define any limits for personality research. Rather, the research leading to the Big Five structure simply constitutes a body of findings too powerful and crucial to be ignored by anyone who seeks to understand human personality. In taking account of this body of findings, it is likely, and appropriate, that the Big Five will be incorporated into a variety of theoretical perspectives (e.g., Buss, Chapter 6, this volume; Tellegen, 1993; Wiggins & Trapnell, in press). The Big Five model is not a threat to other research traditions so much as important information for scientists to utilize. We believe that more than one view can illuminate a subject matter (Shweder, 1989), and that "no doors should be closed in the study of personality" (Allport, 1946, pp. 133–134). We can be more specific about some doors that clearly should be left open.

G. *As a representation of phenotypes based on the natural language, the Big Five structure is indifferent and thus complementary to genotypic representations of causes, motivations, and internal personality dynamics.* The Big Five are dimensions of *perceived* personality. These natural-language dimensions roughly parallel those proposed as a causal model of personality structure by McCrae and Costa (Chapter 3, this volume). This general confluence of everyday person-perception and the constructs in an expert-defined system underlines points we have made earlier: As is the case for physical differences, the natural language is a useful starting point for scientific research on psychological differences; indeed, many other technical classifications have developed from vernacular ones (Simpson, 1961). Personality measurement is unlikely ever to become totally divorced from socially meaningful folk concepts. Nonetheless, folk concepts can be distinguished from formal psychological concepts, even when the latter are relatively close to the former (Tellegen, 1993).

As stated initially by Norman (1963), "It is explicitly *not* assumed that complete theories of personality will simply emerge automatically from such taxonomic efforts. . . . There is a good deal more to theory construction and refinement than the development of an observation language—even a good one" (p. 574). And, as noted more recently by Ozer and Reise (1994), the Big Five model "provides a useful taxonomy, a hierarchical coordinate system, for mapping personality variables. The model is not a theory; it organizes phenomena to be explained by theory" (pp. 360–361).

Delineating the structure of personality attributes is a considerable accomplishment, but this structure implies little about internal personality dynamics or about underlying motivations. Optimally, such dynamics and motivations should be articulated with the Big Five model, and their understanding may be informed by it, but they are in no way determined by it. A point made earlier bears repeating: A model of attributes should not be confused with a model of causal traits. The Big Five is a descriptive rather than an explanatory model. Thus, doors should be left open for explanatory models of all varieties.

Moreover, the Big Five model, like the lexical perspective from which it springs, relies on the person-perception expertise of aggregates of laypersons. As Block (1995) has pointed out, there are other grounds for expertise. Clinicians, teachers, probation officers, scholars of personality psychology—any of these groups could arguably be better judges of personality structure and dynamics than the aggregate layperson, and their perceptions might go well outside and beyond the Big Five model. The lexical perspective and the Big Five model are not inherently incompatible with any of these concerns and perspectives. The lexical perspective can be considered a complement rather than a competitor to other productive streams of personality research. Perhaps one day all the streams may run together into a complete scientific model of personality, but that day is not yet at hand.

In the interim, those who would ignore the contribution already being made by the lexical perspective do so at their own peril. Ozer and Reise (1994) warn us: "Personality psychologists who continue to employ their preferred measure without locating it within the five-factor model can only be likened to geographers who issue reports of new lands but refuse to locate them on a map for others to find" (p. 361).

Acknowledgments

Work on this chapter was supported by Grant No. MH-49227 from the National Institute of Mental Health, U.S. Public Health Service. We are grateful to Hans Eysenck, Sarah Hampson, Willem K. B. Hofstee, Clarence McCormick, Dean Peabody, and Auke Tellegen for their thoughtful comments and suggestions.

Notes

1. Although assumed to be only moderate rather than perfect, the correspondence between lexical representation and substantive importance is the linchpin of the lexical hypothesis, so it is important to consider how it might be shown to be wrong. Relevant would be any investigation that

identifies a broad major personality distinction that has little or no lexical representation, or—even more powerful—any investigation indicating that a lexically emphasized distinction is of no real importance outside language. Also relevant would be any investigation indicating the failure of a previous application of the lexical rationale. For example, Miller and Johnson-Laird (1976) analyzed the semantic properties of verbs and prepositions and identified as psychologically important the following features that are implicit in the lexicon: (1) three-dimensional spatial understanding; (2) a spatialized comprehension of time; (3) among the human senses a central role for vision and a peripheral role for smell and taste; and (4) movement, possession, sensing, and saying as key processes in human life. Could such conclusions be overturned? Probably not without great difficulty. An easier, but less ambitious test of the hypothesis would be an investigation of gross historical changes in the lexicon, as related to important historical changes in human life as recognized through other data sources.

2. One way to index the diachronic life of a descriptive term is by reference to a dictionary of word histories. From the entries in Barnhart (1988) indicating the first-referenced year of their use as person descriptors, it is apparent that a majority of a large set of common personality-related adjectives have seen use in person description for at least 400 years.

3. The difference between nouns denoting objects and nouns identifying single properties is readily illustrated: "The liar lives in the house next door" sounds more awkward than "The man who lives next door is a liar"; the reason is that "liar" is a noun performing an adjective function, meaning "dishonest person," whereas "man" functions as a noun denoting a kind of entity that combines many features. Personality-type nouns such as "liar" probably also differ from nouns denoting objects in lacking the clear hierarchical (genus–species) structure discernible among most of the latter kind of nouns.

4. One class that might prove useful for some purposes are those intransitive verbs that have clear-cut personality implications, such as *talk, fret, laugh,* and *cry.* Such verbs can be used in a sentence frame such as "Compared to others of the same sex and age, the target person *verbs* (1) far less, (2) somewhat less, (3) about the same, (4) somewhat more, or (5) far more than do others." However, such verbs share with their adjectival equivalents the problem of delimiting "personality-relevant" terms from the larger set that includes other person-related variables such as physical and medical descriptors (e.g., *sneeze, cough, drool*) and other types of tangential descriptors (e.g., *kiss, exercise, wash*).

5. The emphasis on factor analysis over cluster-analytic procedures is natural, given a documented linguistic principle (Deese, 1965): Nouns are primarily associated with one another by a grouping scheme (e.g., *crow, raven, blackbird*) that suggests clusters without bipolar relations. However, adjectives are more often associated with one another by a contrast scheme that includes antonyms and bipolarity (e.g., *kind* and *cruel, smart* and *stupid*).

The only adjectives that do not follow this principle seem to be those for color. Because factor analysis can organize variables with bipolar dimensionality, factoring procedures are generally better suited than clustering techniques to analyses of personality-related adjectives.

6. In our view, the cross-language replications of the Big Five model constitute more powerful evidence in its support than do the classic analyses of Tupes and Christal (1961) and others using Cattell's variable selections. Although initially influenced by the lexical hypothesis, Cattell's procedures deviated significantly from the lexical approach; for a review, see John (1990).

7. Most of these terms are used to describe individual differences in political (e.g., *democratic, patriotic, progressive, ultraconservative*) and religious (e.g., *atheistic, irreligious, pious, puritanical*) attitudes.

References

Allport, G. W. (1937). *Personality: A psychological interpretation.* New York: Holt.

Allport, G. W. (1946). Personalistic psychology as science: A reply. *Psychological Review, 53,* 132–135.

Allport, G. W. (1961). *Pattern and growth in personality.* New York: Holt, Rinehart & Winston.

Allport, G. W., & Odbert, H. S. (1936). Trait-names: A psycho-lexical study. *Psychological Monographs, 47*(1, Whole No. 211).

Angleitner, A., Ostendorf, F., & John, O. P. (1990). Towards a taxonomy of personality descriptors in German: A psycho-lexical study. *European Journal of Personality, 4,* 89–118.

Austin, J. L. (1957). A plea for excuses. *Proceedings of the Aristotelian Society, 57,* 1–30.

Bakan, D. (1966). *The duality of human existence.* Boston: Beacon.

Barnhart, R. K. (Ed.). (1988). *The Barnhart dictionary of etymology.* New York: Wilson.

Block, J. (1995). A contrarian view of the five-factor approach to personality description. *Psychological Bulletin, 117,* 187–215.

Block, J. H., & Block, J. (1980). The role of ego-control and ego-resiliency in the organization of behavior. In W. A. Collins (Ed.), *Minnesota symposia on child psychology* (Vol. 13, pp. 39–101). Hillsdale, NJ: Erlbaum.

Brokken, F. B. (1978). *The language of personality.* Meppel, Netherlands: Krips.

Cattell, R. B. (1943). The description of personality: Basic traits resolved into clusters. *Journal of Abnormal and Social Psychology, 38,* 476–506.

Cattell, R. B. (1957). *Personality and motivation: Structure and measurement.* Yonkers, NY: World Book.

Chaplin, W. F., John, O. P., & Goldberg, L. R. (1988). Conceptions of states and traits: Dimensional attributes with ideals as prototypes. *Journal of Personality and Social Psychology, 54,* 541–557.

Chomsky, N. (1957). *Syntactic structures.* The Hague: Mouton.

Costa, P. T., Jr., & McCrae, R. R. (1976). Age differences in personality structure: A cluster-analytic approach. *Journal of Gerontology, 31,* 564–570.

Costa, P. T., & McCrae, R. R. (1992). *Revised NEO Personality Inventory (NEO-PI-R) and NEO Five-Factor Inventory (NEO-FFI) professional manual.* Odessa, FL: Psychological Assessment Resources.

Croft, W. (1991). *Syntactic categories and grammatical relations: The cognitive organization of information.* Chicago: University of Chicago Press.

De Raad, B., & Hofstee, W. K. B. (1993). A circumplex approach to the Five Factor model: A facet structure of trait adjectives supplemented by trait verbs. *Personality and Individual Differences, 15,* 493–505.

De Raad, B., & Hoskens, M. (1990). Personality-descriptive nouns. *European Journal of Personality, 4,* 131–146.

De Raad, B., Mulder, E., Kloosterman, K., & Hofstee, W. K. B. (1988). Personality-descriptive verbs. *European Journal of Personality, 2,* 81–96.

De Raad, B., & Szirmak, Z. (1994). The search for the "Big Five" in a non-Indo-European language: The Hungarian trait structure and its relationship to the EPQ and the PTS. *European Review of Applied Psychology, 44,* 17–26.

Deese, J. (1965). *The structure of associations in language and thought.* Baltimore, MD: Johns Hopkins Press.

Dixon, R. M. W. (1977). Where have all the adjectives gone? *Studies in Language, 1,* 19–80.

Einhorn, H. J., & Hogarth, R. M. (1978). Confidence in judgment: Persistence of the illusion of validity. *Psychological Review, 85,* 395–416.

Eysenck, H. J. (1991). Dimensions of personality: 16, 5, or 3?—Criteria for a taxonomic paradigm. *Personality and Individual Differences, 12,* 773–790.

Goldberg, L. R. (1981). Language and individual differences: The search for universals in personality lexicons. In L. Wheeler (Ed.), *Review of personality and social psychology* (Vol. 2, pp. 141–165). Beverly Hills, CA: Sage.

Goldberg, L. R. (1982). From Ace to Zombie: Some explorations in the language of personality. In C. D. Spielberger & J. N. Butcher (Eds.), *Advances in personality assessment* (Vol. 1, pp. 203–234). Hillsdale, NJ: Erlbaum.

Goldberg, L. R. (1990). An alternative "Description of personality": The Big-Five factor structure. *Journal of Personality and Social Psychology, 59,* 1216–1229.

Goldberg, L. R. (1992). The development of markers for the Big-Five factor structure. *Psychological Assessment, 4,* 26–42.

Goldberg, L. R. (1993a). Author's reactions to the six comments. *American Psychologist, 48,* 1303–1304

Goldberg, L. R. (1993b). The structure of personality traits: Vertical and horizontal aspects. In D. C. Funder, R. D. Parke, C. Tomlinson-Keasey, &

K. Widaman (Eds.), *Studying lives through time: Personality and development* (pp. 169–188). Washington, DC: American Psychological Association.

Goldberg, L. R. (1993c). The structure of phenotypic personality traits. *American Psychologist, 48,* 26–34.

Goldberg, L. R. (1994). How not to whip a straw dog: A critique of Pervin's "Critical analysis of current trait theory." *Psychological Inquiry, 5,* 128–130.

Goldberg, L. R., & Digman, J. M. (1994). Revealing structure in the data: Principles of exploratory factor analysis. In S. Strack & M. Lorr (Eds.), *Differentiating normal and abnormal personality* (pp. 216–242). New York: Springer.

Goldberg, L. R., & Kilkowski, J. M. (1985). The prediction of semantic consistency in self-descriptions: Characteristics of persons and of terms that affect the consistency of responses to synonym and antonym pairs. *Journal of Personality and Social Psychology, 48,* 82–98.

Goldberg, L. R., & Rosolack, T. K. (1994). The Big-Five factor structure as an integrative framework: An empirical comparison with Eysenck's P-E-N model. In C. F. Halverson, G. A. Kohnstamm, & R. P. Martin (Eds.), *The developing structure of temperament and personality from infancy to adulthood* (pp. 7–35). Hillsdale, NJ: Erlbaum.

Goldberg, L. R., & Saucier, G. (1994). So what do you propose we use instead? A reply to Block. *Psychological Bulletin, 117,* 221–225.

Greenwood, J. D. (1991). *Relations and representations.* London: Routledge.

Hampson, S. E. (1994). The construction of personality. In A. M. Colman (Ed.), *Companion encyclopedia of psychology* (pp. 602–621). London: Routledge.

Hampson, S. E., John, O. P., & Goldberg, L. R. (1986). Category breadth and hierarchical structure in personality: Studies of asymmetries in judgments of trait implications. *Journal of Personality and Social Psychology, 51,* 37–54.

Hofstee, W. K. B., & De Raad, B. (1991). Persoonlijkheidsstructuur: de AB5C taxonomie van Nederlandse eigenschapstermen [Personality structure: The AB5C taxonomy of Dutch trait terms]. *Nederlands Tijdschrift voor de Psychologie, 46,* 262–274.

Hofstee, W. K. B., De Raad, B., & Goldberg, L. R. (1992). Integration of the Big Five and circumplex approaches to trait structure. *Journal of Personality and Social Psychology, 63,* 146–163.

John, O. P. (1990). The "Big Five" factor taxonomy: Dimensions of personality in the natural language and in questionnaires. In L. Pervin (Ed.), *Handbook of personality: Theory and research* (pp. 66–100). New York: Guilford Press.

John, O. P., Hampson, S. E., & Goldberg, L. R. (1991). The basic level in personality-trait hierarchies: Studies of trait use and accessibility in different contexts. *Journal of Personality and Social Psychology, 60,* 348–361.

John, O. P., & Robins, R. W. (1993). Gordon Allport: Father and critic of the five-factor model. In K. H. Craik, R. Hogan, & R. N. Wolfe (Eds.), *Fifty years of personality psychology* (pp. 215–236). New York: Plenum Press.

John, O. P., & Robins, R. W. (1994). Traits and types, dynamics and development: No doors should be closed in the study of personality. *Psychological Inquiry, 5,* 137–142.

Kelley, H. H. (1992). Common-sense psychology and scientific psychology. In M. R. Rosenzweig & L. W. Porter (Eds.), *Annual review of psychology* (Vol. 43, pp. 1–23). Palo Alto, CA: Annual Reviews.

Kiss, G. R. (1973). Grammatical word classes: A learning process and its simulation. In G. H. Bower (Ed.), *The psychology of learning and motivation: Advances in research and theory* (Vol. 7, pp. 1–41). New York: Academic Press.

Klages, L. (1926). *Die Grundlagen der Charakterkunde* [*The science of character*]. Leipzig: Barth.

Macnamara, J. (1972). Cognitive basis of language learning in infants. *Psychological Review, 79,* 1–13.

McCrae, R. R. (1990). Traits and trait names: How well is Openness represented in natural languages? *European Journal of Personality, 4,* 119–129.

McCrae, R. R., & Costa, P. T. (in press). Conceptions and correlates of openness to experience. In R. Hogan, J. A. Johnson, & S. R. Briggs (Eds.), *Handbook of personality psychology.* Orlando, FL: Academic Press.

McCrae, R. R., & John, O. P. (1992). An introduction to the five-factor model and its applications. *Journal of Personality, 60,* 175–215.

Miller, G. A., & Johnson-Laird, P. N. (1976). *Language and perception.* Cambridge, MA: Harvard University Press.

Norman, W. T. (1963). Toward an adequate taxonomy of personality attributes: Replicated factor structure in peer nomination personality ratings. *Journal of Abnormal and Social Psychology, 66,* 574–583.

Norman, W. T. (1967). *2800 personality trait descriptors: Normative operative characteristics for a university population.* Unpublished manuscript, Department of Psychology, University of Michigan.

Ostendorf, F. (1990). *Sprache und Persoenlichkeitsstruktur: zur Validitaet des Funf-Faktoren-Modells der Persoenlichkeit* [*Language and personality structure: On the validity of the five-factor model of personality*]. Regensburg, Germany: S. Roderer Verlag.

Ozer, D. J., & Reise, S. P. (1994). Personality assessment. In L. W. Porter & M. R. Rosenzweig (Eds.), *Annual review of psychology* (Vol. 45, pp. 357–388). Palo Alto, CA: Annual Reviews.

Paivio, A., & Begg, I. (1981). *Psychology of language.* Englewood Cliffs, NJ: Prentice-Hall.

Paunonen, S. (1993, August). *Sense, nonsense, and the Big Five factors of personality.* Paper presented at the 101st annual meeting of the American Psychological Association, Toronto, Canada.

Peabody, D. (1987). Selecting representative trait adjectives. *Journal of Personality and Social Psychology, 52,* 59–71.

Peabody, D., & Goldberg, L. R. (1989). Some determinants of factor structures from personality-trait descriptors. *Journal of Personality and Social Psychology, 57*, 552–567.

Pervin, L. A. (1994). A critical analysis of current trait theory. *Psychological Inquiry, 5*, 103–113.

Rosch, E. H., & Mervis, C. B. (1975). Family resemblances: Studies in the internal structure of categories. *Cognitive Psychology, 7*, 573–605.

Ross, L. (1977). The intuitive psychologist and his short-comings. In L. Berkowitz (Ed.), *Advances in experimental social psychology* (Vol. 10, pp. 174–220). New York: Academic Press.

Saucier, G. (1992a). Benchmarks: Integrating affective and interpersonal circles with the Big-Five personality factors. *Journal of Personality and Social Psychology, 62*, 1025–1035.

Saucier, G. (1992b). Openness versus Intellect: Much ado about nothing? *European Journal of Personality, 6*, 381–386.

Saucier, G. (1994a). Mini-markers: A brief version of Goldberg's unipolar Big-Five markers. *Journal of Personality Assessment, 63*, 506–516.

Saucier, G. (1994b, August). *Positive and negative valence: Beyond the Big Five?* Paper presented at the 102nd annual meeting of the American Psychological Association, Los Angeles, CA.

Saucier, G. (1994c). Separating description and evaluation in the structure of personality attributes. *Journal of Personality and Social Psychology, 66*, 141–154.

Saucier, G. (1995, August). *Sampling the latent structure of person descriptors.* Paper presented at the 103rd annual meeting of the American Psychological Association, New York, NY.

Saussure, F. de (1983). *Cours de linguistique générale [Course in general linguistics].* Paris: Payot.

Shadel, W. G., & Cervone, D. (1993). The Big Five versus nobody? *American Psychologist, 48*, 1300–1302.

Shweder, R. A. (1989). Post-Nietzschean anthropology: The idea of multiple objective worlds. In M. Krausz (Ed.), *Relativism: Interpretation and confrontation* (pp. 99–139). Notre Dame, IN: Notre Dame University Press.

Simpson, G. (1961). *Principles of animal taxonomy.* New York: Columbia University Press.

Stagner, R. (1994). Traits and theoreticians. *Psychological Inquiry, 5*, 166–168.

Sternberg, R. J., Conway, B. E., Ketron, J. L., & Bernstein, M. (1981). People's conceptions of intelligence. *Journal of Personality and Social Psychology, 41*, 37–55.

Szirmak, S., & De Raad, B. (1994). Taxonomy and structure of Hungarian personality traits. *European Journal of Personality, 8*, 95–117.

Tellegen, A. (1993). Folk-concepts and psychological concepts of personality and personality disorder. *Psychological Inquiry, 4*, 122–130.

Tellegen, A., & Waller, N. G. (1987, August). *Re-examining basic dimensions of natural language trait descriptors.* Paper presented at the 95th annual meeting of the American Psychological Association, New York, NY.

Tupes, E. C., & Christal, R. E. (1961). *Recurrent personality factors based on trait ratings* (USAF ASD Tech. Rep. No. 61–97). Lackland Air Force Base, TX: U.S. Air Force. (Republished in *Journal of Personality*, 1992, *60*, 225–251)

Tversky, A., & Kahneman, D. (1974). Judgment under uncertainty: Heuristics and biases. *Science, 185*, 1124–1131.

Waller, N. G. (in press). Evaluating the structure of personality. In C. R. Cloninger (Ed.), *Personality and psychopathology*. Washington, DC: American Psychiatric Press.

Whorf, B. L. (1956). *Language, thought, and reality*. New York: Wiley.

Wierzbicka, A. (1986). What's in a noun? (Or: How do nouns differ in meaning from adjectives?) *Studies in Language, 10*, 353–389.

Wiggins, J. S. (1991). Agency and communion as conceptual coordinates for the understanding and measurement of interpersonal behavior. In W. M. Grove & D. Cicchetti (Eds), *Thinking clearly about psychology: Essays in honor of Paul E. Meehl: Vol. 2. Personality and psychopathology* (pp. 89–113). Minneapolis: University of Minnesota Press.

Wiggins, J. S., & Trapnell, P. D. (in press). Personality structure: The return of the Big Five. In R. Hogan, J. A. Johnson, & S. R. Briggs (Eds.), *Handbook of personality psychology*. Orlando, FL: Academic Press.

Wittgenstein, L. (1953). *Philosophical investigations* (G. E. M. Anscombe, Trans.). New York: Macmillan.

Zipf, G. K. (1949). *Human behavior and the principle of least effort*. Cambridge, MA: Addison-Wesley.

Toward a New Generation of Personality Theories: Theoretical Contexts for the Five-Factor Model

ROBERT R. McCRAE
PAUL T. COSTA, JR.

Classic personality theories continue to command the attention of textbook writers and students because contemporary personality research has not made explicit an intellectually satisfying alternative. To move in that direction, we examine in this chapter three theoretical contexts for the five-factor model (FFM): its underlying assumptions of variability, proactivity, rationality, and scientific knowability; its substantive links to individual differences identified in a variety of classic personality theories; and its place within a broad metatheoretical framework for understanding the person. The resulting five-factor theory of personality may serve as a prototype for a new generation of personality theories.

The Lure and Limitations of Personality Theory

When our research was first cited in a major personality theories textbook (Maddi, 1980) it was a heady experience: How thrilling to be mentioned on the same pages as Freud, Allport, and Rogers! Over the next decade, as the FFM grew in prominence in personality research, we noted with great satisfaction that many personality texts devoted some attention to it (e.g., McAdams, 1990a), and were delighted when Pervin (1993) administered our instrument, the NEO Personality Inventory (NEO-PI; Costa & McCrae, 1985, 1989), to the case study he uses to illustrate approaches to personality. Personality texts are, after all, the first introduction that most students have to the field, and those of us who subsequently became personality psychologists naturally cherish the books that first revealed to us our future career.

But as the novelty of citation wore off, we began to adopt a more critical view of personality theory texts, which failed, in our view, to keep pace with progress in the field. It was one thing to share pages with Freud and Allport, but why crowd out contemporary research with accounts of such theorists as Rank and Sheldon? We were disturbed by the charge (see Little, 1989, footnote 6) that our research and that of other advocates of the FFM was "dust bowl" empiricism, by implication inherently inferior to truly theoretical treatments of personality. Why should conceptually grounded research be thought of less merit than the armchair speculations that constitute so much of the history of personality theory?

Mendelsohn (1993) has recently published an impassioned critique of the Theories of Personality enshrined in contemporary texts, documenting their shaky empirical foundation, growing obsolescence, and questionable heuristic value for research in personality. He argued that such theories should be reserved (as they are in other disciplines) for courses in the history of psychology and suggested that personality teachers should introduce their students to contemporary thinking about personality—to share with them the issues that concern academic psychologists in their role as active researchers rather than as intellectual archivists.

At the same time, Mendelsohn acknowledged that "much of the empirical literature is empty and trivial" (p. 113). This theme was emphasized in the same volume by Maddi (1993), who pointed to the fragmentation, overspecialization, and lack of cumulative progress in personality psychology in the wake of the decline of personality theorizing. For Maddi, a comparative analysis of grand theories offers the best hope for integrating psychology into a meaningful science.

These tensions between our loyalties to classic theories and our largely negative scientific evaluation of them, between our commitment to empirical facts and our need for large-scale conceptual frameworks, have pervaded the field of personality psychology for decades, and the resulting paralysis has left a widening gap between textbook introductions to personality psychology and the work that personality psychologists actually do. Mendelsohn's remedy is to abandon the old theories in favor of research. A few textbooks have tried this approach (e.g., Brody, 1972) with limited success. It has become increasingly clear to us that the old theories cannot simply be abandoned: They must be replaced by a new generation of theories that grow out of the conceptual insights of the past and the empirical findings of contemporary research.

A New Beginning for Personality Psychology

If there is a single reason why personality texts have clung so tenaciously to armchair theories, it is the failure of personality researchers until quite recently to provide a compelling alternative. Instead of a coherent body of data supporting one or a few empirical models, researchers generated dozens of minitheories and disputed such elementary questions as the validity of self-report data and the number of basic dimensions of personality (if any). A few empirically oriented theorists (such as Cattell and Eysenck) are represented among the traditional theorists, but after decades of dispute, their differences did not seem any more amenable to empirical resolution than those between other theorists. Mischel's (1968) critique was merely the *coup de grâce* for a long-troubled field.

But much has changed in the past quarter century. The most celebrated empirical accomplishment is the widespread acceptance of the five-factor model as a serviceable description of the structure of personality traits (Digman, 1990; Goldberg, 1993; McCrae, 1992). But there have also been advances in conceptualization and methodology, including the debunking of social desirability as a serious threat to self-report methods (Nicholson & Hogan, 1990) and an appreciation of replicability as the basic criterion for choosing among alternative statistical models (Everett, 1983). Even more fundamental is basic research on personality traits themselves, establishing their heritability (Loehlin, 1992), universality (Yik & Bond, 1993), consensual validation (Funder, 1993), longitudinal stability (Costa & McCrae, 1994), and utility in many applied contexts (e.g., Barrick & Mount, 1991; Miller, 1991). These findings together amount to compelling empirical support for one of the oldest of grand theories of personality, differential psychology (Stern, 1900):

Universal human nature can be understood in terms of enduring individual differences in personality traits.

Research on other aspects of personality has also progressed, although perhaps not as dramatically. We know much more today than we did 25 years ago about the structure and function of the self-concept (Marsh, Barnes, & Hocevar, 1985; Markus & Nurius, 1986), the evolutionary basis of sexual behavior (D. M. Buss, 1989; Simpson & Gangestad, 1992), daily functioning and personal projects (Little, 1983; Tennen, Suls, & Affleck, 1991), unconscious processes and hypnotizability (Kihlstrom, 1987; Roche & McConkey, 1990), autobiography and life narrative (McAdams & Ochberg, 1988), and disorders of personality (Costa & Widiger, 1994; Strack & Lorr, 1994). Such studies demonstrate the continuing vitality of personality research.

Few of these studies originated in tests of classical theories of personality, but none was designed in a conceptual vacuum. The original impetus for the present book was the editor's conviction that theoretical perspectives on the FFM (Wiggins & Trapnell, in press) were unappreciated—a concern shared by McCrae and John (1992), who discussed theoretical implications of the model at some length. At a minimum, the present volume ought to demonstrate that the FFM is not the product of mindless empiricism, but a rich conceptual system that is relevant to many of the central issues raised by classic personality theories.

But a more ambitious goal is possible. Perhaps the time has come to "abandon the course in Theories of Personality" (p. 114) as Mendelsohn (1993) urged and replace historical surveys with contemporary treatments of personality psychology that integrate general frameworks, insightful conceptualizations, and empirical findings. The FFM cannot single-handedly replace the grand theories of personality, because it describes only one aspect of the person. It can however, form the nucleus for a theory of personality that might serve as a model for a new generation of empirically based theories.

Three Functions of Personality Theories

We will not persuade personality psychologists to abandon classic theories until we can offer a better alternative. Such an alternative must self-consciously assimilate the conceptual legacy of the traditional theories, recognizing their contributions to the field. It must also serve the functions of grand theories in organizing knowledge about personality and putting it in broad perspective. Midlevel theories have not shown themselves to be satisfying alternatives to grand theories; what we need are new grand theories.

Personality theories appear to serve three functions. First, they serve as a vehicle for addressing basic philosophical questions about human nature. Psychoanalysis is not merely a school of psychology; it is an intellectual tradition that has profoundly affected literature, the arts, laws, and customs. It had this effect because it proposed a radically new view of human nature. The schools that sprang up in opposition to psychoanalysis were motivated not primarily by disconfirming data, but by different philosophical premises. Much of the power of grand theories comes from their willingness to address these basic, if only quasi-scientific, issues. We will discuss variability, proactivity, rationality, and scientific knowability as fundamental aspects of human nature that are implicit in trait theory and the FFM.

Second, personality theories serve as a repository for insights about psychological mechanisms and human characteristics. Almost all the classic theories include a discussion of individual differences, from Jung's (1971/1923) types to A. H. Buss and Plomin's (1975) temperaments. Measures of many of these constructs have been developed, and one major line of research has linked these theory-based measures to the dimensions of the FFM. Despite its origins in lexical studies, the FFM is not merely a categorization of natural-language trait terms; it is also an organization of constructs articulated by some of our discipline's foremost thinkers.

Finally, at a more abstract level, personality theories define the scope and limits of personality psychology, identifying the variables to be studied and the phenomena to be explained. They direct the attention of the investigator to important questions and provide a standard against which progress in the field can be measured. Without such guidance, explicit or implicit, empirical research is indeed empty and trivial.

Unfortunately, existing personality theories as a body do not give any coherent view of the field. At the end of an introductory course, students do not know whether they should be concerned about dreams, or conditioned responses, or personal constructs, or motives, or identities. The legacy of grand theories at this level is not a unified framework for the study of personality, but a collection of elements or topics, some emphasized in one theory, some in another, like parts of the elephant described by blind men.

We recently offered a model incorporating many of the key elements in personality theories as a basis for distinguishing among definitions of personality (Costa & McCrae, 1994). This model can be seen as a metatheoretical framework for describing personality, identifying the categories of variables that a complete theory of personality ought to address. Existing theories can be compared in this framework, and new theories might be constructed using it as a guide. As an illustration, we sketch a theory built around research on the FFM. We regard this not as a finished product, but as a rough prototype of the next generation of personality theories.

Human Nature and the Five-Factor Model

Hjelle and Ziegler (1976) identified a series of contrasting positions on human nature that they used to compare personality theories. An adaptation of their scheme suggests four basic assumptions that characterize the FFM. The assumptions are generally implicit rather than explicit, but they can be discerned in some form in the entire research enterprise from which the model emerged. Conversely, the empirical success of the FFM provides support for the utility of these assumptions, leading not to a radically new image of human nature but to a restoration of what Brand, Egan, and Deary (1993) called "classical notions of personhood" (p. 224).

Substantive Premises: Variability and Proactivity

As McCrae and John (1992) noted, the FFM is a version of trait theory,[1] a view of human nature with roots in folk concepts (McCrae, Costa, & Piedmont, 1993), Western philosophy (Brand et al., 1993; Costa & McCrae, 1995b), and the pioneering scientific psychology of Sir Francis Galton. Although it has had a continuing influence on personality psychology (A. H. Buss, 1989), trait psychology has always been the stepchild of personality theories. Maddi (1980), for example, relegated the discussion of traits to the periphery of theorizing, and the great paradigm clashes in personality are usually depicted as occurring between psychoanalytic, behavioral, and humanistic traditions. Trait psychology seems dull by comparison.

But trait psychology—supported as it is by abundant empirical data—has profound implications for an understanding of human nature. Personality theory courses are popular in part because they address some very basic philosophical issues: Are we free to chart our own destiny, or are we slaves to our history and culture? Are human beings basically altruistic and trustworthy or fundamentally selfish and manipulative? Must people be forced to work by extrinsic rewards and punishments, or is the achievement of goals intrinsically rewarding? These questions are by no means academic; the answers given to them shape economic systems, legal and religious codes of conduct, and methods of childrearing and education.

To all such questions about the nature of human nature, trait psychology offers a single yet powerful answer: It varies. Some people are independent, some conforming; some are selfish, some generous; some hardworking, some lazy. Any economic system or legal code or childrearing practice that does not make allowances for individual differences will perforce be less than optimal. Snyder (1993), for example, has noted that attempts to motivate prosocial behavior need to take into account the different functions it may serve for different individuals. It is astounding how often this simple principle is ignored. Psychologists are aware of Trait × Treatment interactions (Tellegen, 1981), but they are not routinely studied or implemented even in such familiar contexts as psychotherapy (Miller, 1991). Legislators and social planners are even less likely to make allowances for individual differences.

In part, this may be due to the additional complexity of taking into account individual variation, but in part, it is also due to the bewildering array of individual differences that psychologists have identified over the years. One of the chief merits of the FFM is that it offers a comprehensive yet manageable guide to personality traits. People have individuality, but they are not unfathomably unique. The common trait dimensions of the FFM make variability comprehensible.

Trait psychology makes another basic statement about human nature by seeking the origins of behavior in the individual, implicitly attributing proactivity to the person. Personality traits may have genetic or environmental origins (Plomin & Daniels, 1987; Tellegen et al., 1988), but whatever their source, once established they characterize the individual, not the situation. Sophisticated personality psychologists have never claimed that traits determine behavior independently of situational context (Tellegen, 1991), but they do claim a prominent role for forces within the person as part of the explanation of behavior. In this respect, they assert limits to behavioral, social psychological, and environmental explanations (cf. Costa, McCrae, & Zonderman, 1987).

Intrapersonal determinants of behavior are manifest in some degree of consistency across situations and over time. Wiggins and Trapnell (in press) characterized ours as an "enduring dispositional" approach to the FFM, noting that our findings were based on longitudinal studies of adults. In fact, our belief in dispositions deeply rooted in the individual preceded our adoption of the FFM by several years. In the mid-1970s, when we were obliged to take seriously the possibility that traits might be mere cognitive fictions, the finding of 10-year retest correlations as high as .74 (Costa & McCrae, 1978) was eye-opening. Such data were hard to reconcile with the then-prevalent view that personality was reactive, easily reshaped by social roles, life events, or midlife transitions.

Subsequent evidence on the consensual validation (e.g., Costa & McCrae, 1992c; McCrae, 1982) and predictive utility (e.g., Mutén, 1991; Barrick & Mount, 1991), as well as the long-term stability (Costa & McCrae, 1992c; McCrae & Costa, 1990) of the five factors has nurtured our conviction that individuals are aptly characterized by a distinctive personality-trait profile that shapes their thoughts, feelings, and actions throughout their adult lives. Individuals mention many of these traits spontaneously when asked to respond to the query, "Who am I?" (McCrae & Costa, 1988a); traits thus form an explicit part of their self-concept, providing them with both a sense of uniqueness in comparison with others and a sense of coherence across time. When critics ask where the person is in personality psychology (Carlson, 1984), we believe we speak for our subjects in asserting that much of it is to be found in the proactive dispositions summarized by the FFM.

Methodological Premises:
Scientific Knowability and Rationality

The FFM did not emerge from studies of inkblot responses or experiments on conditioned reflexes or analyses of life narratives. It is the product of factor analyses of personality descriptions obtained from self-reports and observer ratings. As a theory of personality, the FFM is based on a commitment to rigorous quantitative science and an assumption of human rationality. These features distinguish it in important ways from other theories of personality.

From Galton's scatterplots and regression lines to modern item response theory (e.g., Waller & Reise, 1989), trait psychology has been closely allied with psychometrics. Psychometrics, in turn, is a vast mathematical and conceptual structure that is arguably the 20th century's greatest contribution to social science. Even the homeliest scale is likely to incorporate such principles as a standardized response format and aggregation across multiple items, and contemporary measures of the FFM (e.g., Costa & McCrae, 1992b) are evaluated in terms of the replicability of factor structure, retest reliability and stability, and convergent and discriminant validity. Intelligently applied, these psychometric tools give trait psychology a scientific rigor that psychoanalysis has never approached and existential and humanistic theories have frequently disdained.

Behavioral, social learning, and cognitive theories of personality share with trait theories the view that personality can be understood through an application of scientific methods, and Cervone (1991) identified trait/dispositional and social cognitive theories as the "two disciplines" of contemporary personality psychology. One of the major tasks of a new generation of personality theories will be an integration of these two.

Theories of personality differ in assumptions about human rationality. Rationality implies that people generally understand themselves and those around them and act in ways that are consistent with their conscious beliefs and desires. Both radical behaviorism and psychoanalysis are characterized by a rejection of this commonsense view of human nature and by a concomitant rejection of self-reports as a source of data. By contrast, the use of personality questionnaires in research on the FFM carries with it the implication that people are rational.

Most personality questionnaires are rational in the sense that they ask respondents directly to describe themselves, and interpret the responses more or less literally. Even theorists who adopt purely empirical strategies for scale construction generally interpret the scale in terms of item content (Gough, 1965)—a tacit admission of the rationality of respondents. Other researchers prefer scales created by factor analysis, yet factors are almost invariably interpreted by a rational examination of the defining variables.

There is empirical as well as theoretical support for the premise of rationality in questionnaire responses. Hase and Goldberg's (1967) classic comparison of different methods of scale construction found that rational scales performed as well as scales created by other methods. The NEO-PI began with rationally constructed sets of items; item factor analyses confirmed as well as refined these rational groupings; and subsequent research has shown that the resulting scales discriminate such defined groups as patients in psychotherapy and antisocial drug abusers from normal volunteers (Brooner, Schmidt, & Herbst, 1994; Miller, 1991). Accumulating evidence has pointed to the value and accuracy of self-reports (Funder, 1993; Shrauger & Osberg, 1981) and to the utility of straightforward, even transparent, measures (Wolfe, 1993). Individuals are knowledgeable and intelligent observers of their own thoughts, feelings, and behaviors, and thus one excellent source of personality data.

But psychologists who believe in human rationality need not utilize self-reports as their source of data. Observer ratings of traits have the advantage of utilizing the powerful inferential capacities of human judges (Block, 1981) while sidestepping potential falsification or distortion in self-reports. Historically, the FFM was originally uncovered in analyses of peer ratings (Tupes & Christal, 1961/1992), and the Revised NEO-PI (NEO-PI-R) has a validated observer rating form (Costa & McCrae, 1992b).

One of the key pieces of evidence in support of the FFM is the convergence among lay-observer ratings and between observer ratings and self-reports on both the structure of personality traits and the standing of individuals on trait dimensions (McCrae, 1982; Costa & McCrae, 1992c). Expert ratings (McCrae, Costa, & Busch, 1986) and behavioral observations (Funder & Sneed, 1993) provide further support for the model, and thus for the meaningfulness of self-reports and lay ratings.

The fact that individuals know themselves and the people around them well enough to serve as sources of scientific data is testimony to the basic rationality of human nature and to the continuity of folk and scientific conceptions of personality. We would not suggest that folk concepts are fully equivalent to psychological constructs (Tellegen & Waller, in press), or that common sense is a sufficient basis for scientific psychology (Bogdan, 1991; Greenwood, 1991). But we do believe that human beings have a much more sophisticated understanding of human nature than they are sometimes credited with, and that a mature theory of personality need not—indeed, should not—be counterintuitive.

Theory-Based Individual Differences
and the Five-Factor Model

The tenets of variability, proactivity, scientific knowability, and rationality are basic to trait psychology itself, as applicable to the three-factor theory of Eysenck and the 10-factor theory of Guilford as to the FFM. The distinctive feature of the FFM is its claim that it provides a comprehensive system, a framework for organizing virtually all personality traits. Evaluating this claim brings the FFM face-to-face with the body of research based on theories of personality.

It is easy to see that a comprehensive framework would be of enormous utility in guiding systematic research, but it is less easy to see how a model could attain or demonstrate comprehensiveness. One approach to comprehensiveness begins with the fundamental premise of rationality, which asserts that people have at least an implicit understanding of personality. If so, they must also have a language to describe personality. The lexical hypothesis makes the further assumption that personality traits are so central to social interactions in daily life that names for all traits will have been encoded in the language. The laborious work of cataloging all traits can then be assigned to lexicographers, and personality psychologists can concentrate on organizing the finite group of trait-descriptive adjectives in the dictionary. Although strong forms of the lexical hypothesis ("There is a one-to-one correspondence between personality traits and natural-language trait terms") are hard to justify (McCrae, 1990), weaker forms ("Trait terms provide a reasonable guide to a broad range of traits") have worked very well, forming the original basis for the discovery of the FFM (John, Angleitner, & Ostendorf, 1988).

The major objection to lexical studies is that they depend too heavily on commonsense approaches to personality, neglecting the contributions of decades of personality theory and research. Personality scales have been developed to measure most of the important individual differences identified by personality theories; would an analysis of this body of scales also yield the five factors, or would it show that scientific theory has discovered dimensions of personality unknown to laypersons?

Over the past decade, a number of researchers have pursued a systematic analysis of major personality questionnaires in terms of the FFM. These correlational studies have been a vehicle for addressing fundamental conceptual issues such as the relation between needs and traits (Costa & McCrae, 1988) and the validity of typological systems (McCrae & Costa, 1989a), and they have provided the basis for integrative conceptual analyses of the factors (e.g., Costa, McCrae, & Dembroski, 1989; McCrae & Costa, in press). Some of these studies are listed in Table 3.1; as a body, they appear to support three conclusions:

1. Despite diverse theoretical origins, the FFM appears to capture the major dimensions of personality common to most personality scales. The two axes of the Interpersonal Circumplex correspond to Extraversion and Agreeableness; measures of psychopathology are strongly related to Neuroticism. Dachowski (1987) regarded similarities between four of the FFM dimensions and Jungian types as the basis for a convergence between tough- and tender-minded psychologists. Occasional scales (e.g., Thinking Disorder from the Basic Personality Inventory; Jackson, 1989) and factors (e.g., Physical Attractiveness in the California Q-Set; McCrae et al., 1986) appear to lie outside the five-factor space, but these variables are themselves only marginally related to personality. The success with which the FFM accounts for the variance common to scales derived from widely different theoretical perspectives is the most striking evidence of its comprehensiveness.

2. Conversely, each of the five factors has deep conceptual roots in the psychological literature. Consider one example: Conscientiousness. The studies in Table 3.1 show that this factor is related to needs for achievement, order, and endurance, to a judging rather than perceiving cognitive style, to factor-analytic scales measuring superego strength and orderliness, to obsessive–compulsive versus antisocial personality disorders, to temperamental persistence and restraint, and to the use of reason as a tactic of manipulation. The psychological literature thus provides a rich source of conceptualizations for specific facets of each of the five domains (Costa & McCrae, 1995a; Costa, McCrae, & Dye, 1991).

3. A further implication is that traits themselves must be understood from a variety of theoretical perspectives. Some writers (e.g., Pervin, 1994) construe traits narrowly as consistencies in overt behavior—a definition that reduces traits to superficial habits. The studies cited in Table 3.1 suggest that traits are far more complex psychological structures, with cognitive, interpersonal, motivational, and stylistic aspects, some adaptive, some pathological. The FFM is a

TABLE 3.1. Theoretical Perspectives on Some Individual Differences Measured by the Five-Factor Model

Theoretical perspective	Instrument	Convergence with five-factor model
Motivational	PRF (Jackson, 1984)	Borkenau & Ostendorf (1989)
	ACL (Gough & Heilbrun, 1983)	Piedmont, McCrae, & Costa (1991)
	EPPS (Edwards, 1959)	Piedmont, McCrae, & Costa (1992)
Interpersonal	IAS-R (Wiggins, Trapnell, & Phillips, 1988)	McCrae & Costa (1989b)
	ISI (Lorr, 1986)	Lorr, Youniss, & Kluth (1992)
Typological	MBTI (Myers & McCaulley, 1985)	McCrae & Costa (1989a)
Folk conceptual	CPI (Gough, 1987)	McCrae, Costa, & Piedmont (1993)
Factor-analytic	16 PF (Cattell, Eber, & Tatsuoka, 1970)	Gerbing & Tuley (1991)
	EPQ (Eysenck & Eysenck, 1975)	Goldberg & Rosolack (1994)
	CPS (Comrey, 1970)	Boyle (1989)
Psychopathological	MMPI PD (Morey, Waugh, & Blashfield, 1985)	Wiggins & Pincus (1989)
	PDQ-R (Hyler & Reider, 1987)	Trull (1992)
	PAI (Morey, 1991)	Costa & McCrae (1992a)
Temperamental	EASI-III (A. H. Buss & Plomin, 1975)	Angleitner & Ostendorf (1994)
	GZTS (Guilford, Zimmerman, & Guilford, 1976)	McCrae (1989)
Evolutionary	Manipulation tactics	D. M. Buss (1992)
Cross-cultural	Filipino scales	Church & Katigbak (1989)
	Indigenous Chinese scales	Fung Yi Liu (1991)

Note. PRF, Personality Research Form; ACL, Adjective Check List; EPPS, Edwards Personal Preference Schedule; IAS-R, Revised Interpersonal Adjective Scales; ISI, Interpersonal Style Inventory; MBTI, Myers–Briggs Type Indicator; CPI, California Psychological Inventory; 16 PF, Sixteen Personality Factor Questionnaire; EPQ, Eysenck Personality Questionnaire; MMPI PD, Minnesota Multiphasic Personality Inventory Personality Disorder scales; PDQ-R, Revised Personality Disorder Questionnaire; PAI, Personality Assessment Inventory; EASI-III, Emotionality–Activity–Sociability–Impulsivity III; GZTS, Guilford–Zimmerman Temperament Survey.

powerful tool for integrating these different levels of personality functioning in a cohesive description of the individual.

By now, enough theory-based questionnaires[2] have been sampled to allow us to conclude with reasonable certainty that the FFM is indeed comprehensive. The continuing value of studies relating the FFM to other systems is in deepening conceptualization of the five factors and in reconceptualizing other systems. Cartwight and Mori (1988), for example, created the Feelings, Reactions, and Beliefs Survey (FRBS) to measure aspects of the person from a Rogerian perspective. Rogers' (1961) conception of openness to experience played a role in our own initial conceptualization of this dimension (McCrae & Costa, 1985), so it was gratifying, if not surprising, to find that FRBS scales measuring Trust in Self as an Organism and Openness to Transcendental Experiences loaded with an adjective measure of Openness in a joint factor analysis (Cartwright & Peckar, 1993). More interesting was the finding that each of the five factors was defined by at least one of the FRBS scales—for example, the Fully Functioning Person scale was a measure of low Neuroticism. It appears that all five factors are necessary to describe individual differences important in Rogerian theory.

One of the major shortcomings of classical theories of personality is that they often seem to address entirely different aspects of the person, avoiding the constructive confrontations that characterize theorizing in other sciences. The FFM resolves this problem in part by showing how apparently dissimilar constructs are in fact related. What Adler (1938/1964) called *social interest* is akin to what Erikson (1950) called *basic trust* and to what Horney (1945) called *moving toward*—all are aspects of Agreeableness. Explaining the interrelations among these constructs should lead to a deeper understanding of each of the theories. In summary, the FFM provides an empirical synthesis of individual differences identified by personality theories that invites a corresponding conceptual synthesis.

A Metatheoretical Framework
for Personality Theories

We believe that the FFM has a sufficiently strong empirical basis to make it an indispensable aspect of any future theory of personality. People have traits that can be assessed through self-reports or ratings;

that are stable in adulthood; that affect patterns of thought, feeling, and action; and that are organized into five broad dimensions. Standing on these factors is as basic to the description of a person as age, sex, and education, and no personality psychologist can afford to ignore them.

At the same time, we are fully prepared to admit that personality psychologists have been concerned with many aspects of human nature beyond enduring dispositions, and we agree with commentators who note that the FFM does not and cannot provide a complete model of personality (McAdams, 1992; Pervin, 1994). In itself, the FFM does not explain how social roles are forged into a personal identity, or how the flow of behavior is organized, or how attitudes are formed and changed. Traits in the five domains are relevant to each of these topics, but in ways as yet unspecified. Much more than trait psychology is needed to provide a complete explanation of these and many other important phenomena.

In the remainder of this chapter, we will sketch a metatheoretical framework that seems to encompass most of the aspects of human nature identified by theorists and most of the variables with which personality theories have been concerned. Every theory must provide *definitions* of its key variables; the framework highlights categories of variables for which such definitions are needed. Then we will illustrate how a theory of personality might be created within this framework by proposing *postulates* that depict relations among the elements. Our postulates will, naturally, reflect our understanding of the FFM and its role in human psychology. We do not pretend that we can provide a comprehensive theory of personality in the space of a few pages, but we hope to illustrate an approach that may lead to a new and more fruitful generation of personality theories in psychology's next century.

Defining the Elements of Personality Theory

Classical personality theories address very different issues. Psychoanalysts are not overconcerned with the prediction of overt behaviors, but consider dreams of great importance. The opposite is true of social learning theorists. Life structure is important to some theorists (Levinson, Darrow, Klein, Levinson, & McKee, 1978), competence to others (White, 1959). A comparative analysis of personality theories (Maddi, 1993) suggests to us that certain topics or categories of variables recur in many different definitions of personality, and thus that complete theories need to address all these elements (Costa & McCrae, 1994).

Figure 3.1 shows boxes that label five of these elements. All personality theories, we contend, can be construed as statements about these elements and their interrelations. Omitted from the figure is a sixth element, *dynamic processes*, which specify the nature of the interactions among the other elements. In a sense, creating a personality theory consists of detailing the content of the boxes and identifying the causal arrows that connect them.

Table 3.2 lists some of the variables that might be specified for each of the five elements. Personality theories differ in the specific content they address and the importance they assign to it. For example, physical characteristics were central to Sheldon's (1944) constitutional theory of personality, but play a minor role in most other theories. Some elements are missing entirely from some theories—in his empty organism model, Skinner (1974) essentially dismissed the category of basic tendencies. Most theories, however, offer some treatment of each element.

Basic tendencies refer to the universal raw material of personality—capacities and dispositions that are generally inferred rather than observed. Basic tendencies may be inherited, imprinted by early

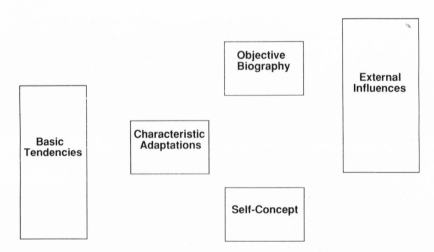

FIGURE 3.1. Categories of personality variables as a metatheoretical framework for personality theories. Adapted from Costa & McCrae (1994).

TABLE 3.2. Examples of Specific Content in Five Categories of Personality Variables

Basic tendencies

Genetics
Physical characteristics
  Sensory–motor capacities
  Health, physical abilities
  Age, race, gender
  Physical appearance
Cognitive capacities
  Perceptual styles
  Operant, respondent learning ability
  General intelligence
    Verbal ability
    Spatial ability
  Specialized talents
Physiological drives
  Needs for oxygen, food
  Sexual drive and orientation
Focal vulnerabilities
  Alcoholism-proneness
  Manic–depressive tendencies

Personality traits
  Neuroticism
    Anxiety, angry hostility, depression
  Extraversion
    Warmth, gregariousness, assertiveness
  Openness to Experience
    Fantasy, aesthetics, feelings
  Agreeableness
    Trust, straightforwardness, altruism
  Conscientiousness
    Competence, order, dutifulness

Characteristic adaptations

Acquired competencies
  Language, general knowledge
  Schemas and strategies
  Social skills
    Etiquette, tactics of manipulation
  Technical skills
Attitudes, beliefs, and goals
  Religious, moral values
  Social, political attitudes
  Tastes, preferences, styles
  Vocational interests
  Personal projects, tasks

(cont.)

TABLE 3.2. (Cont.)

Characteristic adaptations (cont.)

Learned behaviors
  Habits
  Daily routines
  Hobbies
Interpersonal adaptations
  Social roles
  Relationships
  Perceptions of others

Self-concept

Implicit, explicit views of self
Self-esteem
Identity
Life story, personal myth

Objective biography

Overt behavior
Stream of consciousness
Life course
  Career paths
  Historical accidents

External influences

Developmental influences
  Parent–child relations, practices
  Peer socialization
  Education
  Traumatic events
Macroenvironment
  Culture, subculture
  Historical era
  Family, neighborhood, vocational groups
Microenvironment
  Situational constraints
  Social cues
  Motivational press, opportunities
  Reinforcements, punishments

experience, or modified by disease or psychological intervention, but at any given period in the individual's life, they define the individual's potential and direction. Rogers (1961) refers to this aspect of personality as *the organism,* and for many theorists it is the true core of the individual, the real person beneath the mask (Monte, 1977). Jung (1933) would include archetypes; Freud (1933) would add life and death instincts. For us, the most important basic tendencies are personality traits (boxed in the table), construed not as act frequencies (D. M. Buss & Craik, 1983) or consistencies in behavior, but as abstract dispositions.

Characteristic adaptations are acquired skills, habits, attitudes, and relationships that result from the interaction of individual and environment; they are the concrete manifestations of basic tendencies. The full-blooded description of the person that emerges from the personal interview, that stresses current concerns (Klinger, 1977) and interpersonal interactions (Benjamin, 1993), that conditionalizes personality (Thorne, 1989) and emphasizes "doing" rather than "having" (Cantor, 1990) is an account of characteristic adaptations.

The distinction between basic tendencies and characteristic adaptations is crucial to the metatheoretical framework depicted in Figure 3.1; it explains how universal dimensions of personality can exist in widely different cultures, and how "the enduring quality of traits is wholly consistent with the observable changes in behavior that occur with age" (Costa & McCrae, 1980b, p. 90). We have pressed this distinction for years (e.g., McCrae & Costa, 1984; McCrae, 1993a), but have apparently not yet succeeded in making ourselves clear, so a few more words may be in order.

Part of the confusion is semantic. Some writers (e.g., Maddi, 1980; McClelland, 1951) use the term "trait" to refer to specific learned behaviors, "no more than a collection of habits having nothing of the goal-directedness of the motive" (Maddi, 1980, p. 395). Readers with this conception in mind will naturally be puzzled at the inclusion of personality traits among basic tendencies. Like most trait theorists (e.g. Guilford, 1959), we have a different definition of the term "trait" that is much broader and more abstract and clearly includes motivational tendencies (cf. McCrae & John, 1992).

Another part of the confusion is philosophical. Some psychologists are concerned with relatively abstract issues such as the structure of trait adjectives (e.g., Goldberg, 1990) and have little to say about characteristic adaptations. Others (e.g., Cantor et al., 1991) relish the details of personality in living context and have less interest in basic tendencies. There is little reason to bother with the distinction between these two elements if only one is of interest. In our view, personality traits as basic tendencies are the core of personality, but we recognize that they are mere potentialities without their concrete realization in characteristic adaptations.

Finally, part of the confusion is methodological. Questionnaire measures of personality frequently use questions about characteristic adaptations in order to make inferences about basic tendencies. The NEO-PI-R includes items about habits ("I keep my belongings neat and clean"), attitudes ("We can never do too much for the poor and elderly"), relationships ("Most people I know like me"), preferences ("I find philosophical arguments boring"), and social skills ("I don't find it easy to take charge of a situation") in assessing personality traits. It is appropriate to ask about concrete behaviors and preferences because they are signs of the underlying traits, but conceptually they occupy a different level.

Returning to the elements of personality theory shown in Figure 3.1, the *self-concept* consists of knowledge, views, and evaluations of the self, ranging from miscellaneous facts of personal history to the identity that gives a sense of purpose and coherence to life, expressed perhaps in a life narrative or personal myth (McAdams, 1990b, 1993). In one respect, the self-concept is a characteristic adaptation, just as perceptions of others are, but its importance in many theories of personality warrants a separate treatment.

Perhaps the central issue with regard to the self-concept is its accuracy. In psychoanalytic thought, defensive self-deception is ubiquitous. For Rogers, incongruence between the organism and self was psychopathological. Trait psychologists who rely on self-report methods generally assume that the self-concept is reasonably accurate, although they acknowledge that it may sometimes be distorted. Questions about the accuracy of the self-concept arise in the interpretation of longitudinal stability data (McCrae & Costa, 1982) and in the practice of clinical assessment (Costa & McCrae, 1992a).

The *objective biography* consists of "every significant thing that a man [or woman] felt and thought and said and did from the start to the finish of his [or her] life" (Murray & Kluckhohn, 1953, p. 30). The overt behaviors that psychologists observe in laboratories, the dreams that patients recount to their therapists, the fear and joy and anger with which individuals react to life events, and the professional careers that are summarized in obituaries are all aspects of the objective biography. Many theories regard the contents of this category as the outcome variables that personality psychology attempts to predict.

The last element in Figure 3.1 is *external influences*, the psychological environment. Some of the variables in this category are listed in Table 3.2; they include developmental influences and current situations at both the global and specific situational levels. The division of the world into person and environment is, of course, somewhat arbitrary; people help shape the world to which they respond (Bandura, 1989; D. M. Buss, 1987).

Postulating Links: Grand and Midlevel Theories

Many of the postulates of a theory specify relations among the key elements of the theory, and thus correspond to arrows that might be used to connect the boxes in Figure 3.1. These *dynamic processes* bring the model to life, showing paths of development, change, and dynamic equilibrium, and accounting for the ongoing stream of behavior and experience. Some dynamic processes are listed in Table 3.3.

The postulated processes may be very general principles that together form a grand theory of the person, or rather specific

---

TABLE 3.3. Examples of Dynamic Processes in Personality

Information processing
    Preception
    Operant conditioning
    Implicit learning
Coping and defense
    Repression
    Displacement
    Positive thinking
Volition
    Delay of gratification
    Rational choice
    Planning and scheduling
Regulation of emotions
    Emotional reactions (e.g., fight or flight)
    Expression/suppression of affect
    Hedonic adaptation
Interpersonal processes
    Attachment and bonding
    Social manipulation
    Role playing
Identity formation
    Self-discovery
    Search for meaning
    Self-consistency

mechanisms associated with midlevel theorizing. For example, we might postulate broadly that basic tendencies shape characteristic adaptations, or we might attempt to specify precisely *how* tendencies influence adaptations. It was precisely this latter goal that Cantor (1990) addressed in her remarkable attempt to synthesize social cognitive and dispositional approaches. She described "cognitive mechanisms that can mediate the mapping of abstract dispositions onto specific outcomes . . . processes that selectively give form to the blueprint of individuals' personalities" (p. 735).

If the particular mechanisms that Cantor described (notably such strategies as defensive pessimism and self-handicapping) seem rather remote from the traits of the FFM, it is probably because they were developed in a quite different context (cf. Cervone, 1991). In an ideal synthesis, midlevel theories would be generated within the context of a broad theory of personality, which would specify the phenomena to be explained. In the remainder of this chapter, we sketch such a theory, based on research on the FFM. It must be emphasized that this is only one of a large number of personality theories that are compatible with the FFM, but it does illustrate the process and lead to testable predictions. The basic relationships are illustrated in Figure 3.2.

Postulates of a Five-Factor Theory of Personality

1. Basic Tendencies

1a. **Individuality.** *All adults can be characterized by their differential standing on a series of personality traits that influence patterns of thoughts, feelings, and behaviors* (McCrae, 1993b; McCrae & Costa, 1990).

1b. **Origin.** *Personality traits are endogenous basic tendencies.* There is considerable evidence that traits are substantially heritable (Tellegen et al., 1988) but unaffected by shared environmental influences (Plomin & Daniels, 1987); any influence of nonshared environments is hypothetical at this time, and most parsimoniously omitted. Arrows in Figure 3.2 lead out from personality traits, but not in.

1c. **Development.** *Traits develop through childhood and reach mature form in adulthood; thereafter they are stable in cognitively intact individuals.* Data suggest that most traits are fully developed by about age 30 (Costa & McCrae, 1994).

1d. **Structure.** *Traits are organized hierarchically from narrow and specific to broad and general dispositions; Neuroticism, Extraversion, Open-*

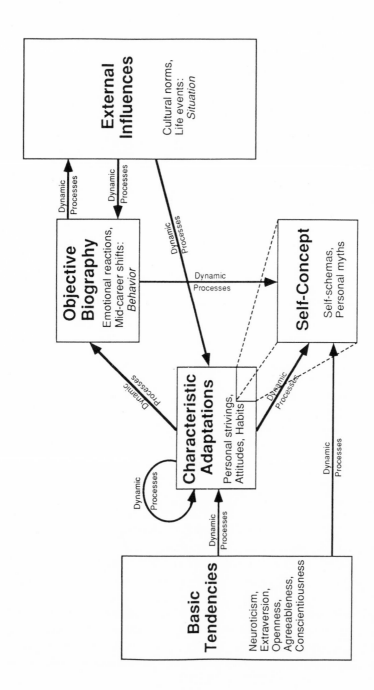

FIGURE 3.2. A five-factor theory of personality, with examples of specific content and arrows indicating the direction of major causal pathways mediated by dynamic processes. Adapted from Costa & McCrae (1994).

ness to Experience, Agreeableness, and Conscientiousness constitute the highest level of the hierarchy (Costa & McCrae, 1995a).

2. Characteristic Adaptations

2a. **Adaptation.** *Over time, individuals react to their environments by evolving patterns of thoughts, feelings, and behaviors that are consistent with their personality traits and earlier adaptations.* Extraverts join social clubs and learn to dance; disagreeable people cultivate cynical attitudes.

2b. **Maladjustment.** *At any one time, adaptations may not be optimal with respect to cultural values or personal goals.* Specifically, when life problems are characteristically related to personality traits, cause significant distress, and are maintained by misperceptions of reality, they can be seen as a *personality-related disorder* (McCrae, 1994).

2c. **Plasticity.** *Characteristic adaptations change over time in response to biological maturation, changes in the environment, or deliberate interventions.*

3. Objective Biography

3a. **Multiple determination.** *Action and experience at any given moment are complex functions of all those characteristic adaptations that are evoked by the situation.* Reading a book utilizes perceptual and cognitive skills and may satisfy an introverted need for solitude, as well as an Openness-related need for intellectual stimulation; there is rarely a one-to-one correspondence between a behavior and a single trait (Ahadi & Diener, 1989).

3b. **Life course.** *Individuals have plans, schedules, and goals that allow action to be organized over long time intervals in ways that are consistent with their personality traits* (cf. Murray & Kluckhohn, 1953).

4. Self-Concept

4a. **Self-schema.** *Individuals maintain a cognitive–affective view of themselves that is accessible to consciousness.* Arrows in Figure 3.2 indicate that the self-concept, itself a specialized subset of characteristic adaptations, reflects aspects of personality traits, other characteristic adaptations, and the objective biography (McCrae & Costa, 1988a).

4b. **Selective perception.** *Information is selectively represented in the self-concept in ways that (i) are consistent with personality traits, and (ii) give a sense of coherence to the individual.*

5. External Influences

5a. **Interaction.** *The social and physical environment interacts with personality dispositions to shape characteristic adaptations and with characteristic adaptations to regulate the flow of behavior.*

5b. **Apperception.** *Individuals attend to and construe the environment in ways that are consistent with their personality traits.*

5c. **Reciprocity.** *Individuals selectively influence the environment to which they respond* (cf. Snyder, 1983). Collectively, individuals create societies and cultures that provide a range of options for expressing personality traits.

6. Dynamic Processes

6a. **Universal dynamics.** *The ongoing functioning of the individual in creating adaptations and expressing them in thoughts, feelings, and behaviors is regulated in part by universal cognitive, affective, and volitional mechanisms.* Perception, learning, planning, and choosing are examples.

6b. **Differential dynamics.** *Some dynamic processes are differentially affected by basic tendencies of the individual, including personality traits.* Open people continue to create new adaptations even when the existing adaptations are adequate; individuals high in Neuroticism emphasize negative information in their self-concepts. All traits are potentially "master traits" that shape the expression of other traits (Costa & McCrae, 1993).

There are probably few surprises in any of these postulates; the basic ideas are familiar from many personality theories, and we have made similar points for years in different contexts. The formal theoretical format, however, makes comparison with other theories easier and places the ideas in a fresh context. Several general comments seem warranted.

The theory ignores universal aspects of personality (Tooby &

Cosmides, 1990) at the level of basic tendencies. It assumes that people live and breathe and move in ways that have evolved to ensure the continuation of their genes. It focuses instead on personality-related individual differences in adaptation. In this respect it resembles Kelly's (1955) "motivationless" theory; indeed, we might adopt as a fundamental postulate a paraphrase of his: *A person's processes are psychologically channelized by his or her standing on the five factors of personality* (p. 46).

Maddi (1980) distinguished three broad classes of personality theories: conflict, fulfillment, and consistency models. Our theory can be classified as a *fulfillment* model, in the sense that personality processes "give form to the blueprint of individuals' personalities" (Cantor, 1990, p. 735). This classification is not immediately obvious, however, because we are accustomed to think of fulfillment in terms of ideal development and specifically to assume that there ought to be concordance between personal and social goals and basic tendencies. Unfortunately, this is not necessarily so. Everyone would like to be rich, but not everyone is willing to work hard; everyone would like to be happy, but not everyone is temperamentally suited to it (Costa & McCrae, 1980a). What all people seem to be able to do with reasonable adequacy is create a life that reflects, for good or ill, their enduring dispositions.

Another important way to characterize theories of personality is in terms of their purpose: What phenomena do they seek to explain and to what questions do they lead the researcher? Personality development is not a major focus of interest, as Postulate 1b makes clear, and Postulate 3a provides little encouragement for predicting specific behaviors. Instead, attention is focused on the prediction of characteristic adaptations—attitudes, interests, roles, lifelong patterns of behavior—personality correlates that constitute the direct and living manifestation of basic dispositions. Understanding exactly how such adaptations evolve is a question of major importance, in part, because it may lead to theories of psychotherapy that promote the development of better adaptations in cases of maladjustment (Miller, 1991).

Finally, it is reasonable to ask how *personality* itself is defined in this theory: Where is personality to be found in Figure 3.2? A tentative answer would identify it with the Basic Tendencies box and its accompanying arrows. Personality consists of a system defined by personality traits and the dynamic processes by which they affect the individual's psychological functioning.

Toward New Theories and New Textbooks

One of the goals of this chapter has been to show that the FFM is not the creation of mindless empiricism, but is instead the product of conceptualizations of personality with rich, if often implicit, theoretical and metatheoretical implications. As Mendelsohn (1993) noted, the "conceptual analysis that both precedes and follows empirical work" (p. 104) is genuine theorizing about personality. In this sense, all the authors in this book are clearly personality theorists.

A more ambitious goal was to help lay the groundwork for a new generation of formal personality theories and textbooks. That will not be accomplished by adding an FFM-based theory to the standard list; instead, it requires the adoption of new attitudes and goals by both personality researchers and textbook writers.

It is easy to criticize textbook authors for perpetuating outmoded theories and neglecting contemporary research, but we must appreciate their role in the field. At one level, personality psychology is an heir to philosophy, claiming to speak with authority on the person as a whole and addressing the great issues of human nature and destiny. It is this aspect of the field that makes it popular with undergraduates and fuels the inspiration of successful textbook authors. (It is probably also this unspoken aspiration in their heart of hearts that distinguishes personality researchers from social psychologists.)

But if personology is to be a science and, in particular, if we are committed to the view that personality is scientifically knowable, then we must insist that answers to the great questions be grounded in empirical data. Classic theories of personality rarely inspire contemporary research, but, as Table 3.1 shows, research on the FFM is relevant to a host of classic theories. For example, our reinterpretation of the Myers–Briggs Type Indicator in terms of the FFM led to a clearly negative evaluation of Jung's typological theory (McCrae & Costa, 1989a). Studies of behavior genetics have wreaked havoc with theories that see parental behaviors as the major source of personality characteristics (McCrae & Costa, 1988b). We now know enough from many sources to eliminate most of the classic theories of personality from further consideration.

But we have not eliminated the need to address the great issues or to put the whole person in a suitably large conceptual framework. New theories are needed, theories that spring from the empirical data rather than the clinician's armchair. The new generation of personality theorists must come from the ranks of personality researchers, those who are willing and able to look up at least occasionally from the midlevel at which they most comfortably function to a higher level that will put their work in a broader perspective.

The five-factor theory of personality we have sketched offers a starting point. As a complete theory it is desperately in need of elaboration, and any psychologists who find it reasonable in broad outline might usefully contribute by detailing the mechanisms by which characteristic adaptations evolve or an integrated life course is constructed (cf. McCrae & John, 1992). Psychologists who take a more critical view of the theory may be stimulated to offer alternatives, drawing different arrows and posing different postulates. Perhaps they can suggest a better general template for personality theories than that described in Figure 3.1 (e.g., Barratt, 1991; Mayer, 1993–1994). But theories of some sort are needed. As the success of the FFM demonstrates, the facts about personality are beginning to fall into place. Now is the time to begin to make sense of them.

Notes

1. This assertion may not accurately characterize the views of Hogan (Chapter 5, this volume) who sees the FFM as a model of social reputations, or of others (e.g., Shweder, 1975), who see the FFM as a model of implicit personality theory. See Borkenau (1992) for a recent evaluation of this latter view.

2. We use the term "questionnaires" advisedly. Projective measures of psychodynamic variables have not yet been systematically related to the FFM, and some studies (Costa & McCrae, 1986; Porter & Rolls, 1992) suggest that few relations will be found. We regard this as further evidence of the limited validity of projective measures (Suinn & Oskamp, 1969).

References

Adler, A. (1964). *Social interest: A challenge to mankind.* New York: Capricorn Books. (Original work published 1938)

Ahadi, S., & Diener, E. (1989). Multiple determinants and effect size. *Journal of Personality and Social Psychology, 56,* 398–406.

Angleitner, A., & Ostendorf, F. (1994). Temperament and the Big Five factors of personality. In C. F. Halverson, G. A. Kohnstamm, & R. P. Martin (Eds.), *The developing structure of temperament and personality from infancy to adulthood* (pp. 69–90). Hillsdale, NJ: Erlbaum.

Bandura, A. (1989). Human agency in social cognitive theory. *American Psychologist, 44,* 1175–1184.

Barratt, E. S. (1991). Measuring and predicting aggression within the context of a personality theory. *Journal of Neuropsychiatry, 3,* S35–S39.

Barrick, M. R., & Mount, M. K. (1991). The Big Five personality dimensions and job performance: A meta-analysis. *Personnel Psychology, 44,* 1–26.

Benjamin, L. S. (1993). *Interpersonal diagnosis and treatment of personality disorders.* New York: Guilford Press.

Block, J. (1981). Some enduring and consequential structures of personality. In A. I. Rabin, J. Aronoff, A. M. Barclay, & R. A. Zucker (Eds.), *Further explorations in personality* (pp. 27–43). New York: Wiley–Interscience.

Bogdan, R. J. (Ed.). (1991). *Mind and common sense: Philosophical essays on commonsense psychology.* Cambridge, UK: Cambridge University Press.

Borkenau, P. (1992). Implicit personality theory and the five-factor model. *Journal of Personality, 60,* 295–327.

Borkenau, P., & Ostendorf, F. (1989). Untersuchungen zum Fünf-Factoren-Modell der Persönlichkeit und seiner diagnostischen Erfassung [Investigations of the five-factor model of personality and its assessment]. *Zeitschrift für Differentielle und Diagnostische Psychologie, 10,* 239–251.

Boyle, G. J. (1989). Re-examination of the major personality-type factors in the Cattell, Comrey and Eysenck scales: Were the factor solutions by Noller et al. optimal? *Personality and Individual Differences, 10,* 1289–1299.

Brand, C., Egan, V., & Deary, I. J. (1993). Personality and general intelligence. In G. L. Van Heck, P. Bonaiuto, I. Deary, & W. Nowack (Eds.), *Personality psychology in Europe* (Vol. 4, pp. 203–228). Lisse, The Netherlands: Swets & Zeitlinger.

Brody, N. (1972). *Personality: Research and theory.* New York: Academic Press.

Brooner, R. K., Schmidt, C. W., Jr., & Herbst, J. H. (1994). Personality trait characteristics of opioid abusers with and without comorbid personality disorders. In P. T. Costa, Jr., & T. A. Widiger (Eds.), *Personality disorders and the five-factor model of personality* (pp. 131–148). Washington, DC: American Psychological Association.

Buss, A. H. (1989). Personality as traits. *American Psychologist, 44,* 1378–1388.

Buss, A. H., & Plomin, R. (1975). *A temperament theory of personality development.* New York: Wiley.

Buss, D. M. (1987). Selection, evocation, and manipulation. *Journal of Personality and Social Psychology, 53,* 1214–1221.

Buss, D. M. (1989). Sex differences in human mate preferences: Evolutionary hypotheses tested in 37 cultures. *Behavioral and Brain Sciences, 12,* 1–49.

Buss, D. M. (1992). Manipulation in close relationships: Five personality factors in interactional context. *Journal of Personality, 60,* 477–499.

Buss, D. M., & Craik, K. H. (1983). The act frequency approach to personality. *Psychological Review, 90,* 105–126.

Cantor, N. (1990). From thought to behavior: "Having" and "doing" in the study of personality and cognition. *American Psychologist, 45,* 735–750.

Cantor, N., Norem, J., Langston, C., Zirkel, S., Fleeson, W., & Cook-Flannagan, C. (1991). Life tasks and daily life experience. *Journal of Personality, 59,* 425–451.

Carlson, R. (1984). What's social about social psychology? Where's the person in personality research? *Journal of Personality and Social Psychology, 47,* 1304–1309.

Cartwright, D., & Mori, C. (1988). Scales for assessing aspects of the person. *Person-Centered Review, 3,* 176–194.

Cartwright, D., & Peckar, H. (1993). Purposefulness: A fourth superfactor? *Personality and Individual Differences, 14,* 547–555.

Cattell, R. B., Eber, H. W., & Tatsuoka, M. M. (1970). *The handbook for the Sixteen Personality Factor Questionnaire.* Champaign, IL: Institute for Personality and Ability Testing.

Cervone, D. (1991). The two disciplines of personality psychology. *Psychological Science, 2,* 371–377.

Church, T. A., & Katigbak, M. S. (1989). Internal, external, and self-report structure of personality in a non-Western culture: An investigation of cross-language and cross-cultural generalizability. *Journal of Personality and Social Psychology, 57,* 857–872.

Comrey, A. L. (1970). *Manual for the Comrey Personality Scales.* San Diego, CA: EdITS.

Costa, P. T., Jr., & McCrae, R. R. (1978). Objective personality assessment. In M. Storandt, I. C. Siegler, & M. F. Elias (Eds.), *The clinical psychology of aging* (pp. 119–143). New York: Plenum Press.

Costa, P. T., Jr., & McCrae, R. R. (1980a). Influence of extraversion and neuroticism on subjective well-being: Happy and unhappy people. *Journal of Personality and Social Psychology, 38,* 668–678.

Costa, P. T., Jr., & McCrae, R. R. (1980b). Still stable after all these years: Personality as a key to some issues in adulthood and old age. In P. B. Baltes & O. G. Brim, Jr. (Eds.), *Life span development and behavior* (Vol. 3, pp. 65–102). New York: Academic Press.

Costa, P. T., Jr., & McCrae, R. R. (1985). *The NEO Personality Inventory manual.* Odessa, FL: Psychological Assessment Resources.

Costa, P. T., Jr., & McCrae, R. R. (1986). Age, personality, and the Holtzman Inkblot Technique. *International Journal of Aging and Human Development, 23,* 115–125.

Costa, P. T., Jr., & McCrae, R. R. (1988). From catalog to classification: Murray's needs and the five-factor model. *Journal of Personality and Social Psychology, 55,* 258–265.

Costa, P. T., Jr., & McCrae, R. R. (1989). *NEO-PI/NEO-FFI manual supplement.* Odessa, FL: Psychological Assessment Resources.

Costa, P. T., Jr., & McCrae, R. R. (1992a). Normal personality assessment in clinical practice: The NEO Personality Inventory. *Psychological Assessment, 4,* 5–13.

Costa, P. T., Jr., & McCrae, R. R. (1992b). *Revised NEO Personality Inventory (NEO-PI-R) and NEO Five-Factor Inventory (NEO-FFI) professional manual.* Odessa, FL: Psychological Assessment Resources.

Costa, P. T., Jr., & McCrae, R. R. (1992c). Trait psychology comes of age. In T. B. Sonderegger (Ed.), *Nebraska symposium on motivation: Psychology and aging* (pp. 169–204). Lincoln: University of Nebraska Press.

Costa, P. T., Jr., & McCrae, R. R. (1993). Ego development and trait models of personality. *Psychological Inquiry, 4,* 20–23.

Costa, P. T., Jr., & McCrae, R. R. (1994). "Set like plaster"? Evidence for the stability of adult personality. In T. Heatherton & J. Weinberger (Eds.), *Can personality change?* (pp. 21–40). Washington, DC: American Psychological Association.

Costa, P. T., Jr., & McCrae, R. R. (1995a). Domains and facets: Hierarchical personality assessment using the Revised NEO Personality Inventory. *Journal of Personality Assessment, 64,* 21–50.

Costa, P. T., Jr., & McCrae, R. R. (1995b). Theories of personality and psychopathology: Approaches derived from philosophy and psychology. In H. I. Kaplan & B. J. Sadock (Eds.), *Comprehensive textbook of psychiatry* (6th ed., Vol. 1, pp. 507–519). Baltimore: Williams & Wilkins.

Costa, P. T., Jr., McCrae, R. R., & Dembroski, T. M. (1989). Agreeableness vs. antagonism: Explication of a potential risk factor for CHD. In A. Siegman & T. M. Dembroski (Eds.), *In search of coronary-prone behavior: Beyond Type A* (pp. 41–63). Hillsdale, NJ: Erlbaum.

Costa, P. T., Jr., McCrae, R. R., & Dye, D. A. (1991). Facet scales for Agreeableness and Conscientiousness: A revision of the NEO Personality Inventory. *Personality and Individual Differences, 12,* 887–898.

Costa, P. T., Jr., McCrae, R. R., & Zonderman, A. B. (1987). Environmental and dispositional influences on well-being: Longitudinal followup of an American national sample. *British Journal of Psychology, 78,* 299–306.

Costa, P. T., Jr., & Widiger, T. A. (Eds.). (1994). *Personality disorders and the five-factor model of personality.* Washington, DC: American Psychological Association.

Dachowski, M. McC. (1987). A convergence of the tender-minded and the tough-minded? *American Psychologist, 42,* 886–887.

Digman, J. M. (1990). Personality structure: Emergence of the five-factor model. *Annual Review of Psychology, 41,* 417–440.

Edwards, A. L. (1959). *Edwards Personal Preference Schedule manual.* New York: Psychological Corporation.

Erikson, E. H. (1950). *Childhood and society.* New York: Norton.

Everett, J. E. (1983). Factor comparability as a means of determining the number of factors and their rotation. *Multivariate Behavioral Research, 18,* 197–218.

Eysenck, H. J., & Eysenck, S. B. G. (1975). *Manual of the Eysenck Personality Questionnaire.* San Diego: EdITS.

Freud, S. (1933). *New introductory lectures in psychoanalysis* (W. J. H. Sprott, Trans.). New York: Norton.

Funder, D. C. (1993). Judgments as data for personality and developmental psychology: Error versus accuracy. In D. Funder, R. Parke, C. Tomlinson-Keasey, & R. Widaman (Eds.), *Studying lives through time: Personality and development* (pp. 121–146). Washington, DC: American Psychological Association.

Funder, D. C., & Sneed, C. D. (1993). Behavioral manifestations of personality: An ecological approach to judgmental accuracy. *Journal of Personality and Social Psychology, 64,* 479–490.

Fung Yi Liu. (1991). *The generalizability of the NEO Personality Inventory to an university sample in Hong Kong.* Unpublished manuscript, Chinese University of Hong Kong.

Gerbing, D. W., & Tuley, M. R. (1991). The 16PF related to the five-factor model of personality: Multiple-indicator measurement versus the a priori scales. *Multivariate Behavioral Research, 26,* 271–289.

Goldberg, L. R. (1990). An alternative "Description of personality": The Big-Five factor structure. *Journal of Personality and Social Psychology, 59,* 1216–1229.

Goldberg, L. R. (1993). The structure of phenotypic personality traits. *American Psychologist, 48,* 26–34.

Goldberg, L. R., & Rosolack, T. K. (1994). The Big Five factor structure as an integrative framework: An empirical comparison with Eysenck's P-E-N model. In C. F. Halverson, G. A. Kohnstamm, & R. P. Martin (Eds.), *The developing structure of temperament and personality from infancy to adulthood* (pp. 7–35). Hillsdale, NJ: Erlbaum.

Gough, H. G. (1965). Conceptual analysis of psychological test scores and other diagnostic variables. *Journal of Abnormal Psychology, 70,* 294–302.

Gough, H. G. (1987). *California Psychological Inventory administrator's guide.* Palo Alto, CA: Consulting Psychologists Press.

Gough, H. G., & Heilbrun, A. B., Jr. (1983). *Adjective Check List manual.* Palo Alto, CA: Consulting Psychologists Press.

Greenwood, J. D. (Ed.). (1991). *The future of folk psychology: Intentionality and cognitive science.* Cambridge, UK: Cambridge University Press.

Guilford, J. P. (1959). *Personality.* New York: McGraw-Hill.

Guilford, J. S., Zimmerman, W. S., & Guilford, J. P. (1976). *The Guilford–Zimmerman Temperament Survey Handbook: Twenty-five years of research and application.* San Diego, CA: EdITS Publishers.

Hase, H. D., & Goldberg, L. R. (1967). The comparative validity of different strategies of deriving personality inventory scales. *Psychological Bulletin, 67,* 231–248.

Hjelle, L. A., & Siegler, D. J. (1976). *Personality: Theories, basic assumptions, research, and applications.* New York: McGraw-Hill.

Horney, K. (1945). *Our inner conflicts.* New York: Norton.

Hyler, S. E., & Rieder, R. O. (1987). *Personality Diagnostic Questionnaire–Revised (PDQ-R).* New York: Author.

Jackson, D. N. (1984). *Personality Research Form manual* (3rd. ed.). Port Huron, MI: Research Psychologists Press.

Jackson, D. N. (1989). *Basic Personality Inventory manual.* Port Huron, MI: Sigma Assessment Systems.

John, O. P., Angleitner, A., & Ostendorf, F. (1988). The lexical approach to personality: A historical review of trait taxonomic research. *European Journal of Personality, 2,* 171-203.

Jung, C. G. (1933). *Modern man in search of a soul* (W. S. Dell & C. F. Baynes, Trans.). New York: Harcourt Brace Jovanovich.

Jung, C. G. (1971). *Psychological types* (H. G. Baynes, Trans.; revised by R. F. C. Hull). Princeton, NJ: Princeton University Press. (Original work published 1923)

Kelly, G. A. (1955). *The psychology of personal constructs* (Vols. 1-3). New York: Norton.

Kihlstrom, J. F. (1987). The cognitive unconscious. *Science, 237,* 1445-1452.

Klinger, E. (1977). *Meaning and void: Inner experience and the incentives in people's lives.* Minneapolis: University of Minnesota Press.

Levinson, D. J., Darrow, C. N., Klein, E. B., Levinson, M. L., & McKee, B. (1978). *The seasons of a man's life.* New York: Knopf.

Little, B. R. (1983). Personal projects: A rationale and method for investigation. *Environment and Behavior, 15,* 273-309.

Little, B. R. (1989). Personal Projects Analysis: Trivial pursuits, magnificent obsessions and the search for coherence. In D. M. Buss & N. Cantor (Eds.), *Personality psychology: Recent trends and emerging directions* (pp. 15-31). New York: Springer-Verlag.

Loehlin, J. C. (1992). *Genes and environment in personality development.* Newbury Park, CA: Sage.

Lorr, M. (1986). *Interpersonal Style Inventory (ISI) manual.* Los Angeles: Western Psychological Services.

Lorr, M., Youniss, R. P., & Kluth, C. (1992). The Interpersonal Style Inventory and the five-factor model. *Journal of Clinical Psychology, 48,* 202-206.

Maddi, S. R. (1980). *Personality theories: A comparative analysis* (4th ed.). Homewood, IL: Dorsey Press.

Maddi, S. R. (1993). The continuing relevance of personality theory. In K. H. Craik, R. Hogan, & R. N. Wolfe (Eds.), *Fifty years of personality psychology* (pp. 85-101). New York: Plenum Press.

Markus, H., & Nurius, P. (1986). Possible selves. *American Psychologist, 41,* 945-969.

Marsh, H. W., Barnes, J., & Hocevar, D. (1985). Self-other agreement on multidimensional self-concept ratings: Factor analysis and multitrait-multimethod analysis. *Journal of Personality and Social Psychology, 49,* 1360-1377.

Mayer, J. D. (1993-1994). A System-Topics framework for the study of personality. *Imagination, Cognition, and Personality, 13,* 99-123.

McAdams, D. P. (1990a). *The person: An introduction to personality psychology.* San Diego, CA: Harcourt Brace Jovanovich.

McAdams, D. P. (1990b). Unity and purpose in human lives: The emergence of identity as a life story. In A. I. Rabin, R. A. Zucker, R. A. Emmons, &

S. Frank (Eds.), *Studying persons and lives* (pp. 148–200). New York: Springer.

McAdams, D. P. (1992). The five-factor model *in* personality: A critical appraisal. *Journal of Personality, 60,* 329–361.

McAdams, D. P. (1993). *The stories we live by: Personal myths and the making of the self.* New York: William Morrow.

McAdams, D. P., & Ochberg, R. L. (Eds.). (1988). Psychobiography and life narratives [Special issue]. *Journal of Personality, 56*(1).

McClelland, D. C. (1951). *Personality.* New York: Dryden.

McCrae, R. R. (1982). Consensual validation of personality traits: Evidence from self-reports and ratings. *Journal of Personality and Social Psychology, 43,* 293–303.

McCrae, R. R. (1989). Why I advocate the five-factor model: Joint analyses of the NEO-PI with other instruments. In D. M. Buss & N. Cantor (Eds.), *Personality psychology: Recent trends and emerging directions* (pp. 237–245). New York: Springer-Verlag.

McCrae, R. R. (1990). Traits and trait names: How well is Openness represented in natural languages? *European Journal of Personality, 4,* 119–129.

McCrae, R. R. (Ed.). (1992). The Five-Factor Model: Issues and applications [Special issue]. *Journal of Personality, 60*(2).

McCrae, R. R. (1993a). Curiouser and curiouser! Modifications to a paradoxical theory of personality coherence. *Psychological Inquiry, 4,* 300–303.

McCrae, R. R. (1993b). Moderated analyses of longitudinal personality stability. *Journal of Personality and Social Psychology, 65,* 577–585.

McCrae, R. R. (1994). Psychopathology from the perspective of the five-factor model. In S. Strack & M. Lorr (Eds.), *Differentiating normal and abnormal personality* (pp. 26–39). New York: Springer.

McCrae, R. R., & Costa, P. T., Jr. (1982). Self-concept and the stability of personality: Cross-sectional comparisons of self-reports and ratings. *Journal of Personality and Social Psychology, 43,* 1282–1292.

McCrae, R. R., & Costa, P. T., Jr. (1984). *Emerging lives, enduring dispositions: Personality in adulthood.* Boston: Little, Brown.

McCrae, R. R., & Costa, P. T., Jr. (1985). Openness to experience. In R. Hogan & W. H. Jones (Eds.), *Perspectives in personality* (Vol. 1, pp. 145–172). Greenwich, CT: JAI Press.

McCrae, R. R., & Costa, P. T., Jr. (1988a). Age, personality, and the spontaneous self-concept. *Journal of Gerontology: Social Sciences, 43,* S177–S185.

McCrae, R. R., & Costa, P. T., Jr. (1988b). Do parental influences matter? A reply to Halverson. *Journal of Personality, 56,* 445–449.

McCrae, R. R., & Costa, P. T., Jr. (1989a). Reinterpreting the Myers–Briggs Type Indicator from the perspective of the five-factor model of personality. *Journal of Personality, 57,* 17–40.

McCrae, R. R., & Costa, P. T., Jr. (1989b). The structure of interpersonal traits: Wiggins's circumplex and the five-factor model. *Journal of Personality and Social Psychology, 56,* 586–595.

McCrae, R. R., & Costa, P. T., Jr. (1990). *Personality in adulthood.* New York: Guilford Press.

McCrae, R. R., & Costa, P. T., Jr. (in press). Conceptions and correlates of Openness to Experience. In R. Hogan, J. A. Johnson, & S. R. Briggs (Eds.), *Handbook of personality psychology.* Orlando, FL: Academic Press.

McCrae, R. R., Costa, P. T., Jr., & Busch, C. M. (1986). Evaluating comprehensiveness in personality systems: The California Q-Set and the five-factor model. *Journal of Personality, 54,* 430–446.

McCrae, R. R., Costa, P. T., Jr., & Piedmont, R. L. (1993). Folk concepts, natural language, and psychological constructs: The California Psychological Inventory and the five-factor model. *Journal of Personality, 61,* 1–26.

McCrae, R. R., & John, O. P. (1992). An introduction to the five-factor model and its applications. *Journal of Personality, 60,* 175–215.

Mendelsohn, G. A. (1993). It's time to put theories of personality in their place, or, Allport and Stagner got it right, why can't we? In K. H. Craik, R. Hogan, & R. N. Wolfe (Eds.), *Fifty years of personality psychology* (pp. 103–115). New York: Plenum Press.

Miller, T. (1991). The psychotherapeutic utility of the five-factor model of personality: A clinician's experience. *Journal of Personality Assessment, 57,* 415–433.

Mischel, W. (1968). *Personality and assessment.* New York: Wiley.

Monte, C. F. (1977). *Beneath the mask: An introduction to theories of personality.* New York: Praeger.

Morey, L. (1991). *Personality Assessment Inventory: Professional manual.* Odessa, FL: Psychological Assessment Resources.

Morey, L. C., Waugh, M. H., & Blashfield, R. K. (1985). MMPI scales for DSM-III personality disorders: Their derivation and correlates. *Journal of Personality Assessment, 49,* 245–251.

Murray, H. A., & Kluckhohn, C. (1953). Outline of a conception of personality. In C. Kluckhohn & H. A. Murray (Eds.), *Personality in nature, society, and culture,* (2nd. ed., pp. 3–52). New York: Knopf.

Mutén, E. (1991). Self-reports, spouse ratings, and psychophysiological assessment in a behavioral medicine program: An application of the five-factor model. *Journal of Personality Assessment, 57,* 449–464.

Myers, I. B., & McCaulley, M. H. (1985). *Manual: A guide to the development and use of the Myers–Briggs Type Indicator.* Palo Alto, CA: Consulting Psychologists Press.

Nicholson, R. A., & Hogan, R. (1990). The construct validity of social desirability. *American Psychologist, 45,* 290–292.

Pervin, L. A. (1993). *Personality: Theory and research* (6th ed.). New York: Wiley.

Pervin, L. A. (1994). A critical analysis of current trait theory. *Psychological Inquiry, 5,* 103–113.

Piedmont, R. L., McCrae, R. R., & Costa, P. T., Jr. (1991). Adjective Check

List scales and the five-factor model. *Journal of Personality and Social Psychology, 60,* 630–637.

Piedmont, R. L., McCrae, R. R., & Costa, P. T., Jr. (1992). An assessment of the Edwards Personal Preference Schedule from the perspective of the five-factor model. *Journal of Personality Assessment, 58,* 67–78.

Plomin, R., & Daniels, D. (1987). Why are children in the same family so different from one another? *Behavioral and Brain Sciences, 10,* 1–16.

Porter, B. J., & Rolls, S. (1992). Personality and perception: Rorschach and Luescher correlates of Jungian types as measured by the Myers–Briggs Type Indicator. In C. D. Spielberger & J. N. Butcher (Eds.), *Advances in personality assessment* (Vol. 9, pp. 117–125). Hillsdale, NJ: Erlbaum.

Roche, S. M., & McConkey, K. M. (1990). Absorption: Nature, assessment, and correlates. *Journal of Personality and Social Psychology, 59,* 91–101.

Rogers, C. R. (1961). *On becoming a person: A therapist's view of psychotherapy.* Boston: Houghton Mifflin.

Sheldon, W. (1944). Constitutional factors in personality. In J. McV. Hunt (Ed.), *Personality and the behavior disorders* (pp. 526–549). New York: Ronald.

Shrauger, J. S., & Osberg, T. M. (1981). The relative accuracy of self-predictions and judgments by others in psychological assessment. *Psychological Bulletin, 90,* 322–351.

Shweder, R. A. (1975). How relevant is an individual difference theory of personality? *Journal of Personality, 43,* 455–484.

Simpson, J. A., & Gangestad, S. W. (1992). Sociosexuality and romantic partner choice. *Journal of Personality, 60,* 31–51.

Skinner, B. F. (1974). *About behaviorism.* New York: Knopf.

Snyder, M. (1983). The influence of individuals on situations: Implications for understanding the links between personality and social behavior. *Journal of Personality, 51,* 497–516.

Snyder, M. (1993). Basic research and practical problems: The promise of a "functional" personality and social psychology. *Personality and Social Psychology Bulletin, 19,* 251–264.

Stern, W. (1900). *Über Psychologie der individuellen Differenzen (Ideen zur einer "differentielle Psychologie") [On the psychology of individual differences (Ideas for a "differential psychology")].* Leipzig: Barth.

Strack, S., & Lorr, M. (Eds.). (1994). *Differentiating normal and abnormal personality.* New York: Springer.

Suinn, R. M., & Oskamp, S. (1969). *The predictive validity of projective measures: A fifteen year evaluative review of research.* Springfield, IL: Thomas.

Tellegen, A. (1981). Practicing the two disciplines for relaxation and enlightenment: Comment on "Role of the feedback signal in electromyograph biofeedback: The relevance of attention" by Qualls and Sheehan. *Journal of Experimental Psychology: General, 110,* 217–226.

Tellegen, A. (1991). Personality traits: Issues of definition, evidence and assessment. In W. M. Grove & D. Cicchetti (Eds.), *Thinking clearly about psychology: Essays in honor of Paul E. Meehl* (Vol. 2, pp. 10–35). Minneapolis: University of Minnesota Press.

Tellegen, A., Lykken, D. T., Bouchard, T. J., Jr., Wilcox, K. J., Segal, N. L., & Rich, S. (1988). Personality similarity in twins reared apart and together. *Journal of Personality and Social Psychology, 54,* 1031–1039.

Tellegen, A., & Waller, N. G. (in press). Exploring personality through test construction: Development of the Multidimensional Personality Questionnaire. In J. Cheek & E. M. Donahue (Eds.), *Handbook of personality inventories.* New York: Plenum Press.

Tennen, H., Suls, J., & Affleck, G. (Eds.). (1991). Personality and daily experience [Special issue]. *Journal of Personality, 59*(3).

Thorne, A. (1989). Conditional patterns, transference, and the coherence of personality across time. In D. M. Buss & N. Cantor (Eds.), *Personality psychology: Recent trends and emerging directions* (pp. 149–159). New York: Springer-Verlag.

Tooby, J., & Cosmides, L. (1990). On the universality of human nature and the uniqueness of the individual: The role of genetics and adaptation. In D. M. Buss (Ed.), Biological foundations of personality: Evolution, behavioral genetics, and psychophysiology [Special issue]. *Journal of Personality, 58,* 17–68.

Trull, T. J. (1992). DSM-III-R personality disorders and the five-factor model of personality: An empirical comparison. *Journal of Abnormal Psychology, 101,* 553–560.

Tupes, E. C., & Christal, R. E. (1992). Recurrent personality factors based on trait ratings. *Journal of Personality, 60,* 225–251. (Original work published 1961)

Waller, N. G., & Reise, S. P. (1989). Computerized adaptive personality assessment: An illustration with the Absorption scale. *Journal of Personality and Social Psychology, 57,* 1051–1058.

White, R. W. (1959). Motivation reconsidered: The concept of competence. *Psychological Review, 66,* 297–333.

Wiggins, J. S., & Pincus, A. L. (1989). Conceptions of personality disorders and dimensions of personality. *Psychological Assessment: A Journal of Consulting and Clinical Psychology, 1,* 305–316.

Wiggins, J. S., & Trapnell, P. D. (in press). Personality structure: The return of the Big Five. In R. Hogan, J. A. Johnson, & S. R. Briggs (Eds.), *Handbook of personality psychology.* Orlando, FL: Academic Press.

Wiggins, J. S., Trapnell, P., & Phillips, N. (1988). Psychometric and geometric characteristics of the Revised Interpersonal Adjective Scales (IAS-R). *Multivariate Behavioral Research, 23,* 119–134.

Wolfe, R. N. (1993). A commonsense approach to personality measurement. In K. H. Craik, R. Hogan, & R. N. Wolfe (Eds.), *Fifty years of personality psychology* (pp. 269–290). New York: Plenum Press.

Yik, M. S. M., & Bond, M. H. (1993). Exploring the dimensions of Chinese person perception with indigenous and imported constructs: Creating a culturally balanced scale. *International Journal of Psychology, 28,* 75–95.

CHAPTER FOUR

A Dyadic–Interactional Perspective on the Five-Factor Model

JERRY S. WIGGINS
PAUL D. TRAPNELL

We cannot doubt that more complex formal systems will eventually
add new spatial dimensions to the organization of personality. For
the present, however, a two-dimensional space offers sufficient
complexity for the data and more than a sufficient complexity of
methodological problems.

—LEARY (1957, p. 64)

In the above characteristically prescient observation, Timothy Leary
summarized the state of the art of circumplex models of interpersonal behavior during the 1950s and anticipated the need for additional spatial dimensions to provide a more comprehensive picture
of personality organization. Although not all methodological problems have been solved since that time, we are currently much more
knowledgeable about the applications of circumplex models to personality data (e.g., Browne, 1992; Wiggins, Steiger, & Gaelick, 1981)
and about the role of that model in theory construction and evaluation (e.g., Gurtman, 1992a; Wiggins, Phillips, & Trapnell, 1989)
than we were in the "pre-Guttman" era during which Leary's observations were made. Moreover, as the chapters in the present book
attest, there is now substantial agreement on the nature of some of
the additional spatial dimensions that are needed to augment the
original circumplex dimensions of Surgency/Extraversion and

Agreeableness: namely, Conscientiousness, Neuroticism, and Intellect/Openness to experience.

The theoretical orientation that we have chosen to call the "dyadic–interactional perspective" (Pincus & Wiggins, 1992; Trapnell & Wiggins, 1990; Wiggins & Pincus, 1994; Wiggins & Trapnell, in press) represents an exceptionally longstanding tradition in personality assessment. The history of this tradition, like that of the equally venerable five-factor model (FFM), has been characterized by extended "interruptions" over time (Craik, 1986) that may be related to concurrent developments in other areas of psychology that occurred during successive epochs (Wiggins, 1985). But the most remarkable feature of the interpersonal tradition has been its resiliency and perdurability in the face of changing conceptualizations and methodological innovations in the fields of personality, social, and clinical psychology.

On the conceptual side, it is not surprising that a theory so deeply rooted in the writings of Harry Stack Sullivan should survive earlier controversies surrounding "interactionism" (Carson, 1989), the nature of social exchange (Carson, 1979), or the currently heavy emphasis on information processing and allied cognitive concepts in personality and social psychology (Carson, 1991). On the methodological side, it may also not be surprising that factor-analytic investigators have begun to discover merit in circumplex models of personality (e.g., Hofstee, De Raad, & Goldberg, 1992). More recent, and more germane to the present chapter, is the increasing realization that the two dimensions that define the universe of content of interpersonal behavior (dominance and nurturance) are rotational variants of the first two dimensions of the FFM (McCrae & Costa, 1989; Trapnell & Wiggins, 1990). Finally, the recently discovered success of the FFM in clarifying psychiatric conceptions of personality disorders in DSM-III-R (Costa & Widiger, 1994) must be attributed in large part to the two circumplex dimensions of that model which stem from a clinical tradition that has already served a similar function for the personality disorders of DSM-I (e.g., Leary, 1957), DSM-II (e.g., Plutchik & Platman, 1977), and DSM-III (e.g., Wiggins, 1982).

The dyadic–interactional view differs from other perspectives on the FFM in the *conceptual priority* assigned to the first two factors of the model and in the *structural model* used to represent those factors. Within the realm of classical theories of personality, our orienting attitudes are perhaps closest to those of Harry Stack Sullivan (1953a) whose field-theoretical unit of observation was the "relatively enduring pattern of recurrent interpersonal situations that characterize a human life" (pp. 110–111). Sullivan also believed in the unity of the social sciences, the value of anthropological investigations of other cultures, and the importance of language and communication for the understanding of interpersonal situations (Cohen, 1953). In this respect, our orientation to the FFM is compatible in a number of ways with Hogan's (1983) sociological theorizing, Goldberg's (1981) emphasis on language and cross-cultural generalizability, and as will be seen with D. M. Buss's (1991b) evolutionary approach to personality.

The conceptual priority accorded to the factors of *dominance* (Surgency/Extraversion) and *nurturance* (Agreeableness) stems from our conviction that these statistical abstractions from personality psychometrics correspond most closely to the immensely broader concepts of agency and communion that pervade the humanities and social sciences, as well as many classical and contemporary theories of personality. In the material that follows, we will illustrate this pervasiveness with examples from evoluntionary, anthropological, sociological, cross-cultural, and narrative life-history perspectives. We next provide a more focused application of the metaconcepts of agency and communion to the social psychological concept of social exchange that is essential to our understanding of the interpersonal dynamics of Factors I and II. This material is followed by a review of interpersonal conceptions of dominance and nurturance and of the measurement procedures employed to capture these concepts. In the final part of this chapter, we consider the three additional factors of the FFM within the conceptual framework provided by the dyadic–interactional perspective.

The Metaconcepts of Agency and Communion

If I am not for myself, who will be for me? But if I am
only for myself, what am I?
                                        —PIRKE AVOT

The terms "agency" and "communion" were adopted by David Bakan (1966) "to characterize two fundamental modalities in the existence of living forms, agency for the existence of an organism as an individual, and communion for the participation of the individual in some larger organism of which the individual is a part" (pp. 14–15).

Although the two concepts are highly abstract, Bakan's essay related them to ordinary human experience and empirical research in a *tour de force* that ranged over such topics as religion, science, myth, sexuality, death, and disease.

In a somewhat more prosaic attempt to relate the concepts of agency and communion to the study of interpersonal behavior, Wiggins (1991a) illustrated the centrality of these concepts to philosophical worldviews from Confucius to Bakan, personality theorists from Freud to McAdams, psycholinguistic and historicodevelopmental studies of the language of personality, and conceptions of men and women, from a variety of disciplines. The following sections augment this earlier survey by considering some of the different guises that the agency–communion distinction has assumed when central issues of different disciplines have been addressed. Table 4.1 provides an overview of this material.

Evolutionary Perspective

Darwin's (1859) theory of natural selection emphasized solutions to adaptive problems of two major kinds: those of survival and those of reproduction. Survival is, of course, a prerequisite to becoming an eventual contributor to future generations, but the specific problems of and solutions to the successful reproduction

TABLE 4.1. Conceptions of Agency and Communion within Different Disciplines

Field	Focus	Agency	Communion
Evolutionary psychology (D. M. Buss, 1991b)	Solution of reproductive problems	Negotiation of status hierarchies	Formation of reciprocal alliances
Anthropology (Redfield, 1960)	Common challenges provided by all societies	Getting a living	Living together
Sociology (Parsons & Bales, 1955)	Divisions of labor within societies	Instrumental roles	Expressive roles
Cross-cultural psychology (Triandis, 1990)	Cultural bases of social behavior among societies	Individualistic societies	Collectivist societies
Narrative life history (McAdams, 1993)	Themes in myth, stories, and individual lives	Power	Love

of progeny tend to be more social in nature and hence more central to the dyadic–interactional viewpoint (D. M. Buss, 1991b, pp. 464–465). With respect to solutions of the latter problems, it is common to speak of *inclusive fitness*, which refers to an individual's reproductive success, together with the individual's influence upon the reproductive success of relatives. *Nota bene* that the notion of inclusive fitness does not assume a general motivation on the part of individuals (conscious or unconscious) to maximize their reproductive success in successive generations, an assumption that D. M. Buss has dubbed the "sociobiological fallacy." Instead, it is assumed that certain anatomical, physiological, and psychological characteristics exist in their present form because they were associated at some time in the dim past with successful solutions of specific adaptive problems of reproduction.

Darwin (1871) based his theory of *sexual selection* on the assumption that members of one sex compete for opportunities to mate with reproductively valuable members of the opposite sex. The nature of this intrasexual competition differs between the sexes, in part because of the differing amounts of *parental investment* in offspring that usually exist between men and women (Trivers, 1972). For example, the cost to women of producing one offspring (as opposed to other offspring) may involve extended periods of gestation and lactation, whereas men, at a minimum, need only provide sperm. Similarly, whereas the reproductive success of women is constrained by the quality and quantity of resources they can secure for themselves and their offspring, the reproductive success of men is constrained primarily by the sheer number of fertile women they can inseminate (D. M. Buss & Schmitt, 1993). These differences between men and women are reflected in sex differences in traits and strategies associated with reproductive success (D. M. Buss, 1994, 1995; Chapter 6, this volume).

Sexual selection can occur because of successful competition with members of one's own sex or because some members of one sex possess characteristics that are appealing to members of the opposite sex (Kenrick, 1989). Intrasexual competition on a social level often assumes an agentic form for men and a communal form for women. Men who are able to successfully negotiate *status hierarchies* have a decidedly competitive advantage (e.g., more resources and better mating opportunities). Women who successfully form *reciprocal alliances* with others have greater access to protection and resources (D. M. Buss, 1986). On the level of intersexual attractiveness, the trait of *dominance* in men is appealing to women (D. M. Buss, 1989; Sadalla, Kenrick, & Vershure, 1987), and social traits associated with *nurturance* in women are appealing to men (D. M. Buss, 1989; Kenrick & Keefe, 1989).

Anthropological Perspective

In a notably clear and succinct chapter on "how society operates," Redfield (1960) observed: "A society is people with common ends getting along with one another" (p. 345). Members of a society work together on their common problems of *getting a living* and *living together*. The anthropological perspective on these enterprises is informed by studies of primitive societies in which the basic elements of social organization can be viewed more clearly than in larger, more complex, and rapidly changing societies.

The enterprise of getting a living requires some degree of specialization, and the divisions of labor between men and women and between the young and the old are universal:

> In some small, isolated, primitive societies there is almost no division of labor except between the sexes and the age-groups, and except some individuals who act as magicians or as leaders of ceremonies. With the development of tools and techniques, with increase in population, and with the advancement of communication and transportation, the division of labor has become far more complete and complex. (Redfield, 1960, p. 346)

A highly differentiated society provides more commodities and services for the populace but makes it more difficult for the average individual to comprehend the overall goals and operations of society as a whole.

The enterprise of living together is facilitated and made more rewarding by the feeling of group solidarity referred to as *esprit de corps*. This sense of belongingness is enhanced by contrasting the members of one's own society with the members of other societies: "Many primitive tribes reserve the term for 'people' or 'human beings' to themselves alone, while everywhere the terms used to refer to neighboring peoples are contemptuous, derogatory" (p. 349). In societies that are divided into subgroups with local loyalties that are subordinated to the interests of the larger society, *esprit de corps* may be increased: "There is a special kind of strength in a tribe divided into clans, for each clan is a warm and supporting intimate group for every individual within it; its limited solidarity is intensified by the contrast and competition with other clans" (p. 349).

Redfield (1960) discusses a third principle of social organization that would seem to underlie both the agentic enterprise of getting a living and the communal experience of living together: "Perhaps the basic form of the organization of work arises from the fact that in a society people share common sentiments and beliefs as to what it is good to do" (p. 347). These "shared convictions about the good life" render work a part of the meaning of life and provide an agreed upon plan of life that defines proper customs and conduct in a "single moral representation of the universe." "The body of conventional meanings that are made known to us through acts and artifacts is by anthropologists called 'the culture' of a community" (p. 347). Only in primitive societies can one see the unitary nature of culture and its influence upon getting a living and living together. "[The peasant's] view of the good life is not much lifted above the horizon of subsistence and persistence, but lifted it is enough to make it possible for later eyes and greater inspiration to cast our human vision far out into the universe" (Redfield, 1962, p. 37).

Sociological Perspective

From a sociological perspective, one can identify agentic and communal themes in the divisions of labor that occur within societies to meet the universal challenges of getting a living and living together. The distinction between *instrumental* and *expressive* roles first made by Parsons and Bales (1955) was influential in advancing this line of thought. The original focus of convenience of these authors' investigations was upon the *sex-role* differentiations that occur within the nuclear family, (and hence the social structures impinging on the developing child). These differentiations may be represented by the two coordinates of function priority (instrumental vs. expressive) and power hierarchy (high vs. low status). To attain the goals of the family (getting things done in the outside world) fathers enact, and socialize their sons toward, roles involving manipulations of the environment. To foster integration and minimize tensions (maintaining harmony within the family) mothers enact, and socialize their daughters toward, roles facilitating and supporting attachments among family members.

As to the contentious issue of why instrumental and expressive roles are assigned to men and women, respectively, Parson and Bales suggest that women's experiences of childbearing and nursing establish a "strong presumptive primacy" for adopting expressive roles and that men, being "exempted from these biological functions," tend to specialize in alternative instrumental directions. Their argument is not basically a biological one, however. From their sociological perspective, Parson and Bales maintain that the instrumental–expressiveness dimension found in the nuclear family is a qualitative dimension that appears in *all* social systems (as exemplified by the small-groups work of Bales, 1950). "Indeed, we argue that probably the importance of the family and its functions for society constitutes the primary set of reasons why there is a *social* as distinguished from purely reproductive, differentiation of sex roles" (Parson & Bales, 1955, p. 22, italics in original).

Parson and Bales view the fourfold structure of roles in the nuclear family as "basic" to the child's eventual understanding of successively more complex social systems outside the family unit. Thus, for example, within a broader societal context the instrumental–expressiveness dimension becomes further differentiated into universalistic and particularistic roles. Instrumental roles of males can be universalistic (technical expert) or particularistic (executive leader); expressive roles of females can be universalistic ("cultural" expert) or particularistic (charismatic leader).[1]

Cross-Cultural Perspective

In a far-reaching and highly integrative chapter on cross-cultural perspectives, Triandis (1990) identified the dimension of *individualism versus collectivism* as "perhaps the most important dimension of cultural difference in social behavior, across the diverse cultures of the world" (p. 42). The importance of this dimension as a focus of cross-cultural study is brought home by the fact that "almost all the data of psychology come from individualistic cultures, yet about 70% of the population of the world lives in collectivist cultures" (p. 48). The shortcomings of this possible ethnocentric bias became even more evident from the results of Triandis's own research. For example, he found that the American definition of "individualism" (self-reliance, competition, and distance from in-groups) contributed only slightly to the variance among cultures of the world, and he commented that "what is most important in the United States is least important worldwide" (p. 50).

Within individualistic cultures, a person's social behavior is best understood as the pursuit of personal goals, the attainment of which benefits individuals. The formulation of personal goals usually occurs without reference to the goals of "collectives" within the culture (e.g., the family, the work group, the state). Should there arise a conflict between personal and group goals, it is generally acceptable to place the former ahead of the latter. Individualistic themes that appear in Western texts stress the dignity of humans, individual self-development, autonomy, privacy, and the individual as the basis of society (Lukes, 1973).

Within collectivist cultures, a person's social behavior is best understood as the pursuit of goals shared with one or more collective, the attainment of which benefits the group. Should there arise a conflict between personal and group goals, the latter are placed ahead of the former. Social scientists agree in characterizing members of collectivist cultures as being concerned about the results of their actions on others, sharing material and nonmaterial resources with group members, being concerned about their presentation to others, believing in the correspondence of outcomes of self and group, and feeling involved in the contributions and sharing in the lives of group members (Hui & Triandis, 1986).

Although societies may be distinguished from one another on the collectivism–individualism dimension, it should be emphasized that these patterns coexist within a given society. Triandis (1990) offers the analogy of the coexistence of *water* (collectivism) and *ice* (individualism) to illustrate this pattern of coexistence. Although young children are highly dependent upon the family at first (collectivism), they eventually become more independent and self-reliant (individualism). Even though collectivist patterns (water) have been transformed to individualist patterns (ice), traces of the former remain and the latter may "melt back" to its origins. In Triandis's analogy, the molecules of ice correspond to particular relationships of the individual with friends, coworkers, and neighbors: "In each culture a different pattern of those self–other links becomes ice. So there are different kinds of individualism and different kinds of collectivism, depending on whether the predominance of the molecules are water or have been transformed into ice" (p. 44).

Triandis, Leung, Villareal, and Clack (1985) made further distinctions between individualism–collectivism at the *cultural* level and idiocentrism–allocentrism at the *individual* level. These distinctions, together with appropriate instruments to measure them, have allowed Triandis to explore both group differences among cultures and individual differences within cultures. Two factors emerged from multivariate analyses of differences among cultures: *Family Integrity* was the best marker of worldwide collectivism (e.g., "Aging parents should live at home with their children") and *Detachment from In-groups* was the best marker of worldwide individualism (e.g., feeling emotionally detached from subgroups within a culture). Two different factors emerged from multivariate analyses of individual differences within cultures: *Interdependence and Sociability* was the best marker of allocentrism within a culture, and *Self-Reliance* was the best marker of idiocentrism (Triandis et al., 1986).

Space limitations preclude summarizing even a portion of the additional empirical work done by Triandis and his coworkers over the last decade (see Triandis, 1995), but some mention should be made of the implications of that work for sex roles that would seem to be compatible with propositions of the evolutionary, anthropological, and sociological perspectives. Triandis (1990) noted the striking parallels that exist between male–female social behavior (Eagly, 1987), male–female relationship difficulties (Gilligan, 1982) and the cross-cultural findings for individualism–collectivism.

Narrative Life-History Perspective

The study of individual lives over time is a topic of investigation in so many different disciplines (e. g., history, literature, psychoanalysis, and most of the social sciences) that one is hard pressed to identify common assumptions and practices (Runyon, 1988). For present purposes, we will focus on mainstream psychobiography in psychology, as represented by the work of Dan McAdams, that has given explicit emphasis to agency and communion as organizing themes in individual life stories (McAdams, 1985a, 1985b, 1989, 1990, 1991, 1993).

McAdams (1993) has articulated a neo-Eriksonian theory of identity development that is enriched by more contemporary concepts such as image, theme, prototype, scripts, and personal myths. The basic premise of his position is that each person creates, consciously or unconsciously, a heroic story of the self, a personal myth that is "a patterned integration of our remembered past, perceived present, and anticipated future" (p. 12). Agency and communion are the two superordinate content themes of such narratives. From a psychological perspective, agency and communion represent the two central motivational clusters in human life: power/achievement and intimacy/love. "Power and achievement . . . share an emphasis on the active assertion of the self over and against the surrounding environment" (p. 72). Intimacy and love are overlapping desires through which "each of us is able to relate to others in warm, close, and supportive ways" (p. 72).

McAdams (1993) describes the origins and development of personal myths within the context of Erikson's (1959) stages of psychosocial development and with an emphasis on the superordinate content themes of agency and communion. During the first stage of development, relationships with parents form the basis of a sense of hope (or despair) in the infant. This, in turn, contributes to the *narrative tone* of later personal myths (optimism vs. pessimism). During the preschool years, children learn the *images* (emotionally charged symbols) of stories available in their culture, and these images eventually become incorporated within their personal myths. During the elementary-school years, children come to understand the intentional and goal-directed nature of stories, and they begin to develop their own patterns of power and intimacy motivation; images become transformed into *themes.*

Like Erikson, McAdams considers the stage of adolescence to be critical to identity formation. It is during the latter part of this period that adolescents become "self-conscious mythmakers," as McAdams puts it. The development of formal operational thinking during this period inclines the adolescent to raise basic questions regarding alternative worlds and to be concerned generally with issues of goodness and truth. It is this context of philosophical rumination that provides the *ideological setting* for the development of future personal myths. Agency and communion are the superordinate themes of the fundamental beliefs and values that provide ideological settings. Agentic ideologies value the autonomy and well-being of the individual over everything else. Communal ideologies value the group and interpersonal relationships most highly. McAdams's (1993) description of the content of agentic and communal ideological settings for personal myths (pp. 87–89) is remarkably similar to Triandis's (1990) summary of the values of individualist and collectivist cultures discussed earlier.

The term "imagoes" was chosen by McAdams (1993) to describe the nature of the main *characters* in life stories: "Imagoes are archetypical patterns for human thought and conduct that compose idealized personifications in personal myth" (p. 124). Elsewhere (McAdams, 1985a), this concept is differentiated from related formulations, such as archetypes (Jung, 1943), personifications (Sullivan, 1953a) internalized objects (Fairbairn, 1952) ego states (Berne, 1972), scripts (Steiner, 1974), prototypes (Cantor & Mischel, 1979), and possible selves (Markus & Nurius, 1986). McAdams's concept of imago is based on an empirically derived taxonomy that is organized in accordance with the metaconcepts of agency and communion, and exemplified by 12 gods and goddesses from ancient Greek mythology. The imago types illustrated by this taxonomy represent prototypes of high agency, high communion, high agency *and* communion, and low agency *and* low communion (McAdams, 1985a, 1985b, 1990, 1993)[2]:

> *The Sage* (Zeus) is a controlling, judgmental, distant figure for whom significant others are either creations or creators of one's own agentic image (high agency).
>
> *The Caregiver* (Demeter) is a nurturant, altruistic, gentle figure for whom significant others are either caregivers or recipients of care (high communion).
>
> *The Peacemaker* (Athene) is a generative, prudent, ambivalent figure whose relationships affirm both agency and communion in the roles of arbiter, counselor, teacher, and guide (high agency *and* communion).

Like any well-told tale, a personal myth emphasizes those dramatic high points, low points, and turning points in a life narrative that are particularly meaningful and important to the main character. In forging a personal identity, we tend to select and reconstruct certain scenes from our past that illustrate either our continuity over time or the beginnings of personal change. McAdams (1993) calls these scenes *nuclear episodes,* and he interprets them in terms of power and intimacy motivation at different stages of ego development. Persons highly motivated by power tend to remember nuclear episodes centered on themes of strength/impact, status/recognition, autonomy/independence, and competence/accomplishment. Persons with high intimacy motivation recall nuclear episodes that stress love/friendship, dialogue/sharing, care/support, and unity/togetherness.

The "ending" of life narratives has the uniquely human quality of being both a termination and a new "beginning" through which the self may live on. This is the essence of the concept of generativity, which Erikson viewed as a discrete stage in the human life cycle, but which McAdams (1993) construes as an evolving personal myth that is continuous from late adolescence onward. The question of generativity arises naturally from the logic and structure of the total life narrative: "The action of the story [*theme*] is situated within a setting of belief and value [*ideological setting*]; the main characters of the story have been established as personified and idealized images of self [*imagoes*]; and the significant story high points, low points, and turning points have been organized as landmark events of the past [*nuclear episodes*]. Given all this, *what is to be done in the future?*" (McAdams, 1985b, p. 252, italics in original).

Generativity, according to McAdams, is a two-step process that involves creating a product (e.g., composing a poem) and "giving up" or offering that product to a community (e.g., publishing the poem). A *generativity script* is a plan of action that outlines what an individual intends to do to ensure that a legacy of him- or herself will be left to the next generation. Because such a script is part of an evolving personal myth, it will be generally compatible with the themes, ideological settings, imagoes, and nuclear episodes that form the other components of that myth.

The empirical research of McAdams (1985b) supports the compatibility of generativity scripts with other components of the personal myth. Subjects who score high on power or intimacy motivation tend to produce generativity scripts emphasizing agentic or communal motivation, respectively. The degree of generativity of a script (concern for establishing and guiding the next generation) was modestly associated with intimacy motivation and slightly associated with power motivation. However, a combined score on intimacy and power motivation proved to be more strongly related to degree of generativity, nicely confirming McAdams's two-step hypothesis regarding generativity: The creation of a product is an agentic enterprise, and the sharing of that product with others is a communal venture; both are required for effective generativity.

The Nature of Social Exchange

Resource Classes

Interpersonal transactions may be thought of as occasions for "exchanges" in which individuals give or take away resources from each

other. This notion has long been intuitively appealing to social philosophers, economists, social psychologists and others who have
sought to characterize the principles governing these exchanges with
concepts such as reciprocity, equity, distributive justice, and complementarity. However, aside from such obvious resources as money and
material goods, the full universe of *content* of social exchange has
seldom been specified with any degree of comprehensiveness (D. M.
Buss & Schmitt, 1993). The notable exception to this lack of specificity may be found in the theory of social exchange proposed by Foa
and Foa (1974, 1976, 1980; Foa, Converse, Törnblom, & Foa, 1993)
that serves as a major conceptual foundation for the dyadic–interactional perspective on personality (Carson, 1969). In particular, we
have employed the Foas' theory to distinguish *interpersonal* events
from other categories of exchange by defining the former as *"dyadic
interactions that have relatively clear-cut social (status) and emotional (love)
consequences for both participants (self and other)"* (Wiggins, 1979, p. 398,
italics in original). Agency and communion are thus identified as the
coins of the realm of interpersonal exchange. There are other ten-
ders that may be offered or withheld, however, and the Foas' cognitive-developmental theory provides an arguably complete taxonomy
of these additional resources and their relations to status and love.

The Foas' taxonomy of resources is based, in part, on assumptions regarding the relative order in which these categories become
meaningful to us in the course of our cognitive development. The
arrows in Figure 4.1 are meant to provide a highly simplified representation of a developmental sequence. Out of the newborn's undifferentiated bundle of *love* and *service* (warmth, softness, food, care), a
distinction between the two resources becomes possible as "self"
becomes distinguished from "other" (e.g., feeding oneself vs. being
fed). Love (acceptance, liking) is eventually differentiated from *status*
(esteem, regard), although the two are closely related (e.g., "I am very
proud of you"). Service becomes differentiated from *goods* when the
concept of object permanence is acquired. Status and *information* also
become differentiated, although the relation between them remains
in such phenomena as "credibility of informational source." Finally,
a distinction is acquired between the similar resources of goods and
money.

The circular configuration of resources in Figure 4.1 is meant to
convey the similarity of *meaning* among resources, in part as a function of the developmental period during which they became differentiated. Resources that became differentiated from one another at a

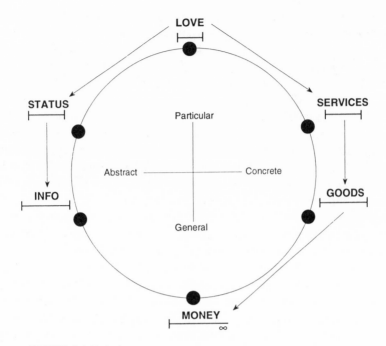

FIGURE 4.1. Relations among resource classes of social exchange.

given developmental stage tend to retain some of their similarities in meaning throughout adult life. The meaning–similarity relations depicted in Figure 4.1 are also predicted to obtain from a structural model that specifies the coordinates of the circular configuration. Specifically, the Foas postulate a horizontal dimension of *concreteness* and a vertical dimension of *particularism* as the underlying coordinates that give rise to a circumplex of social resources.

It is recognized in a number of disciplinary contexts that communications are expressed in forms that vary from the concrete to the symbolic. With respect to the exchange of resources, "Some behaviors, like giving an object or performing an activity upon the body or the belongings of another individual, are quite concrete. Some other forms of expression, such as language, posture of the body, a smile, a gesture, or facial expression, are more symbolic" (Foa & Foa, 1974, p. 81).

In Figure 4.1, it can be seen that performing (or not performing) specific services and giving (or withholding) particular goods are concrete forms of exchange. In contrast, the sharing of information or the granting of status is a more symbolic mode of exchange. In the intermediate range are love, which can be both concrete (a caress) and symbolic (red roses) and money, which can also be both concrete (cash) and symbolic (credit card).

The vertical dimension of particularism "indicates the extent to which the value of a given resource is influenced by the particular persons involved in exchanging it and by their relationship" (p. 80). The distance between love and money on this dimension (Figure 4.1) is easily understood. It is a matter of relative indifference who cashes one's payroll check, but avowals of love from a total stranger are clearly less valuable than those from one's beloved. Similarly, the conferring of status and the offering of services are more appreciated when granted by significant others. In contrast, it is less important *who* provides information and goods and more important that the information be accurate and the goods be of high quality.

Both the developmental order in which resource classes emerge and the underlying coordinates of concreteness and particularism generate quite specific structural hypotheses regarding social exchange: (1) with respect to the *meaning-similarity* of resources, it is hypothesized that the more two resources are proximal in the order, the more they will be perceived as similar; (2) with respect to *resource-exchange,* it is hypothesized that preferences for different resources that might be received in exchange for a resource that has been given will decrease progressively the more the anticipated resources are distal from the most preferred resource to be received; (3) the circumplex patterning of preference for exchange just described will be *invariant,* no matter which resource is given.

Turner, Foa, and Foa (1971) provided data that tended to confirm the three hypotheses just stated. Messages were typed on cards to represent the six resource classes, for example, "I feel affection for you" (love), "Here is my opinion" (information), "Here is some money for you" (money). In testing the meaning-similarity hypothesis, subjects were led to believe that they were receiving a series of messages from a fellow student and were asked to return the "most similar" and the "most dissimilar" messages to the one received. The results for the "most similar" exchanges are presented in Table 4.2. The rows are the resources received from the confederate, and the columns are the messages judged by the subjects to be most similar to the messages they received. The expected circular patterns are indicated by small crosses. Subjects were not given the option of responding to a resource class with a message from that same class (the similarity of messages *within* classes was established in pretests). Although the entries in Table 4.2 are percentages rather than correlations, the pattern is clearly recognizable as a quasi circumplex (Guttman, 1954). Thus, for example, when love is received, similarity decreases to its opposite of money (Figure 4.1) and increases in a circular pattern as love is approached.

Subsequent experiments of a similar nature tended to confirm both the resource–exchange and invariance hypotheses. In social transactions, subjects tend to prefer "exchange in kind," in which "kind" is perceived according to the circumplex shown in Figure 4.1. Thus, if love is given, love is preferred in exchange, followed in decreasing order by status, information, and money (least preferred of all) and in increasing order by goods and services. The invariance of this pattern was established by demonstrating that, in general, a circumplex ordering of preferences for exchange also held when subjects gave each of the other five resource classes to confederates (Turner et al., 1971).

The circumplex representation of resource classes shown in Figure 4.1 may be thought of as comprising fuzzy sets with permeable boundaries that merge indistinguishably into one another (Wiggins, 1980). As the Foas note, we tend to grant status to those we love, value information from high-status sources, appreciate

TABLE 4.2. Percentage of Resource Returned as Being "Most Similar" to Resource Provided

Resource provided	Resource returned					
	Love	Status	Information	Money	Goods	Services
Love		65	10	0	2	23
	++++	++	+	0	+	++
Status	62		20	10	3	5
	++	++++	++	+	0	+
Information	17	34		11	24	14
	+	++	++++	++	+	0
Money	0	16	8		60	16
	0	+	++	++++	++	+
Goods	6	5	21	55		13
	+	0	+	++	++++	++
Services	41	18	7	16	18	
	++	+	0	+	++	++++

Note. Rows sum to 100%. Adapted from Turner, Foa, & Foa (1971, p. 172). Copyright 1971 by the American Psychological Association. Adapted by permission.

affection in restaurants where the "service is good," and so on, with examples that are presumably distributed *continuously* around the circumplex. In principle, one could construct a geometric taxonomy of specific acts and utterances with reference to the angular locations provided by the coordinates of concreteness and particularism, as we have done for particular personality scales (Wiggins & Broughton, 1991). Such a taxonomy would likely bring increased focus to research topics of current interest such as "helping" and "social support."

Social Motives

It is difficult to conceptualize the giving and receiving of resources in social exchange without some rudimentary notion of needs or motives. Within this context, two of the Foas' motivational concepts appear to have the status of metamotives, that is, motives regarding motives: (1) The *need for independence* "represents a wish to have many alternative sources, thus avoiding reliance on any specific individual for obtaining resources"; (2) the *need for security* "indicates a desire to assure *future* supplies of unspecified resources" (Foa & Foa, 1974, p. 130, italics in original). Although not identified as such, these abstract manifestations of agency and communion serve to clarify the social-exchange strategies employed by agentic and communal individuals. It is not the case, for example, that the agentic person is "indifferent" to the resources provided by others; rather, he or she seeks resources in such a way as to avoid being "tied down" to commitments. The communal person, in contrast, is more concerned with "tying down" commitments so as to ensure the future supplies associated with solidarity.

On a less abstract level, the six categories of resources themselves provide a taxonomy of social motives within the Foas' theory. At this level, the concept of the *optimal range* of a motive is especially heuristic. By reasoning similar to that involved in Cannon's (1939) principle of homeostasis and Tomkins's (1965) notion of tolerance limits, the Foas argue that every resource has a lower limit below which motivation is aroused and an upper limit of satiation that varies for different resources. It follows from the latter that each resource has a characteristic optimal range or width of application. This range is indicated by the bracketed lines underneath each resource label in Figure 4.1. Interestingly, love has the smallest optimal range of all resources and, more obviously, money has an almost infinite upper limit. According to the structural ordering, the more particularistic resources of service and status have relatively narrow optimal ranges and the less particularistic resources of goods and services have relatively broad ranges.

Resources with narrow optimal ranges are less stable and are characterized by frequent adjustments. Love, in particular, is an intense and unstable resource. One reason for this is that giving love to another is positively associated with giving love to self and, hence, one does not reduce the amount of love in such exchanges. It is also the case that, unlike money and goods, love cannot be "stored" outside the system. Experiencing a surfeit of love is not uncommon: "We feel miserable being far away from those who love us, but when close to them, we sometimes want to be alone" (Foa & Foa, 1974, p. 129). The Foas further suggest that "lovers' quarrels" may serve a much-needed homeostatic function in reducing the amount of that resource to within tolerable limits. In contrast, the broader optimal-range categories of goods and money are more stable, involve resources that can be easily stored or banked, and result in net loss when given away. Information, on the other side of the circle, can be transmitted without gain or loss to the transmitter, and the granting of status tends to decrease the status of the granter.

The dyadic–interactional perspective on personality emphasizes exchanges involving the particularistic resource classes of love (communion) and status (agency) in close relationships. Love is the most particularistic of resource classes, and it is central to close relationships in both its abstract manifestations that merge with agentic concerns (status) and its more concrete expressions that merge with the provision of services to loved ones. Status, although more general and more abstract, is an equally important component of close relationships that merges with the provision of information to significant others.

As previously mentioned, the exchange of love and status in close relationships involves correlated tendencies between giving to (or taking from) others. Giving love to another typically entails giving love to one's self and thereby results in a net increase of this resource for the giver.[3] This principle has been part of common wisdom for many centuries and is well expressed in Tolstoy's observation: "We do not love people so much for the good they have done us, as for the good we have done them." The Foas have provided empirical confirmation of this principle in many situations and cultures (Foa et al., 1993). The opposite state of affairs exists for the resource of status: Granting status to another typically entails denial of status to self and vice versa. As Wilde put it, "We can forgive anything in a friend but success." This is not surprising, given the ordinary meaning of "status" that connotes a *relative* position on a social hierarchy.

The emphasis of the dyadic–interactional perspective upon the resources of love and status is not meant to imply that these resources are exchanged independently of the other four: "Resources are like chemical elements: in nature, they seldom occur in a pure state, but they provide a basis for classifying and analyzing the compounds they form" (Foa & Foa, 1980, p. 82). The universe of content of social exchange illustrated in Figure 4.1 may be thought of as depicting the inherently *interdisciplinary* context in which the study of interpersonal behavior is embedded. The efforts of other social scientists to include sociological, psychological, political, and economic concepts in models of resource exchange (e.g., Ilchman & Uphoff, 1969) could well be reciprocated by psychologists.

Summary of Conditions for Exchange

Overall, the conditions that facilitate or impede social exchange include (1) the motivational states of potential exchangers; (2) the appropriateness of the environmental or institutional settings in which exchanges take place; and (3) the properties of the specific resources to be exchanged (Foa & Foa, 1974, Chap. 5).

We have already discussed the notion of a lower limit for resources, below which an individual is motivated to seek replenishment, and the idea of an upper limit that varies widely among resources. To these, we add the Foas' concept of *power* which is "the amount of a given resource that is available to an individual for eventual giving" (p. 135). For example, a high-status individual is empowered to expect love from others in exchange for granting them status—provided that others are, in fact, deficient in status. But such power is useless among others who themselves have an optimal level of status. Hence, the ideal exchange situation is one in which "each participant is powerful in the specific resource the other needs" (p. 136).

Opportunities for exchanges among individual who have reciprocal needs and powers are facilitated by social institutions that provide suitable settings for such exchanges: "The exchange of money with services is typical of the work institution; information is exchanged in school institution, if private, and status is exchanged for information in public schools; money–goods exchange is found in the trade institution; and in the family, love and status are the crucial resources" (p. 151). The psychotherapeutic setting may be thought of as a social institution governed by differing rules for the exchange of resources, depending upon the theoretical orientation of the therapist (pp. 152–155). For example, in orthodox psychoanalytic treatment, the patient gives money and information (free associations) to the therapist, who reciprocates with information (interpretations). The patient is expected to give love to the therapist (transference), but reciprocation in kind is discouraged (countertransference); the patient is also expected to grant unreciprocated status to the therapist. In contrast, the counselor in Rogerian therapy grants noncontingent love and status to the client, who is encouraged to grant these to him- or herself.[4]

Among the most distinctive contributions of the Foas to the theory of social exchange is their specification of the many ways in which resource classes systematically differ from one another as a function of their proximity on the two-dimensional circumplex illustrated in Figure 4.1. The cognitive structuring of resource classes within the coordinates of concreteness and particularism results in distinctively different principles of exchange being associated with different resource classes. These differing principles have implications for both the motivational states of potential exchanges (e.g., love can be given to another without loss to self; money given is money lost) and the appropriateness of institutional settings for exchange (e.g., giving and receiving love requires an environment that persists over an extended period of time; money can be exchanged rapidly in short-lived settings).

Interpersonal Conceptions of Personality

I have become occupied with the science, not of individual
differences, but of human identities, or parallels, one might say.
In other words, I try to study the degrees and patterns of things
which I assume to be ubiquitously human.
                                        —SULLIVAN (1953a, p. 33)

Historical Considerations

Elsewhere, Wiggins (1991a) observed that Freud's eventual contribution to the agency–communion framework for understanding personality may have been a negative one; his neglect of the communal domain appears to have been the principal impetus behind the defection of the neo-Freudians (Adler, Horney, Fromm) who, in turn, laid the foundations for such later developments as Erikson's magisterial integration of the individual and society. Table 4.3 provides examples of the manner in which the dual themes of agency and communion have appeared in various guises in personality theories that originated in psychoanalytic, behavioral, and humanistic contexts. Although the ubiquitousness of agentic and communal themes in theories of personality may facilitate the classification and comparison of theories on an abstract level, a more critical issue concerns the basic unit of observation that is adopted to capture these themes. We have found the *interpersonal* unit of observation employed by Sullivan to be the most useful in this respect.

Principle of Communal Existence

From an earlier treatise on biology (Eldridge, 1925), Sullivan (1953a) adopted a principle of communal existence that is meant to apply to all organisms: "The living cannot live when separated from what might be described as their necessary environment" (p. 31). The necessary environment for humans, as contrasted with plants and animals, must include *culture.* "Since culture is an abstraction pertain-

TABLE 4.3. Conceptions of Agency and Communion within Theories of Personality

Theorist	Agency	Communion
Freud (1933/1964)	Able to work	Able to love
Adler (1933/1964)	Striving for superiority	Social interest
Horney (1937)	Moving against others	Moving toward others
Angyal (1941)	Autonomy	Homonomy
Fromm (1941)	Separate entity	Openness with world
Rank (1945)	Individuation	Union
Erikson (1950)	Autonomy	Basic trust
Sullivan (1953)	Self-esteem	Security
Rotter (1954)	Recognition–status	Love and affection
Foa (1965)	Status	Love
Maslow (1971)	Esteem needs	Belongingness and love needs
Hogan (1983)	Achieving status	Maintaining peer popularity
McAdams (1985)	Power motivation	Intimacy motivation

ing to people . . . man requires interpersonal relationships or interchange with others" (p. 32). The verb "requires" is here meant quite literally; to be cut off from interchange with others is, in Sullivan's view, not unlike an animal being cut off from sources of oxygen, in terms of psychological well-being.

Sullivan's account of human motivation employs the familiar distinction between primary (physiological) and secondary (psychogenic) needs, and emphasizes the equally familiar notion of tension (drive) reduction in explaining the acquisition of responses. However, his unique emphasis upon the *interpersonal* nature of needs in the human organism adds a dimension not present in other accounts. Tensions are tendencies toward overt actions, whose aim is to provide satisfaction and return the organism to a state of relative equilibrium. But the meaning (and hence the basis of classification) of these patterns of satisfaction-seeking tendencies is to be found in the behaviors of *other persons* whose "cooperation" is required to provide the satisfaction sought. And the kind and degree of satisfaction received depends heavily upon the existence of "complementary" patterns of motivation in potentially cooperative others. The need for tenderness in the infant and the corresponding need of the mother to provide tenderness serve as the paradigm of this type of exchange. Later, more complex combinations of needs and actions are held to be "interpersonal in kind, if not in all details" (p. 41).

Interpersonal Anxiety

The developing infant's gradual recognition that *survival* depends upon one's "success or failure in bringing about the appearance, approach, and cooperation of the good mother in connection with the satisfaction of a need" (Sullivan, 1953a, p. 92) is accompanied by anxiety. The concept of anxiety is among the most central, and is certainly the most all-inclusive, of the concepts in Sullivan's system. Although Sullivan clearly located the origins of anxiety in the earliest mother–infant relationship, the precise manner whereby the mother "induces" anxiety in the infant was "thoroughly obscure" (p. 41). To bridge this gap in knowledge, Sullivan suggested the use of the undefined term "empathy" to characterize the process whereby the infant detects the mother's anxiety; a suggestion that subsequently was widely criticized, but tenaciously held to by Sullivan: "There is much that sounds mysterious in the universe, only you have got used to it; and perhaps you will get used to empathy" (p. 42).

According to Chapman (1976), the inclusiveness of Sullivan's concept of anxiety may be its most problematic feature: "*By anxiety he means virtually all basic types of emotional suffering.* . . . It perhaps would have been better if Sullivan had employed a different term to designate so broad a spectrum of painful feelings" (p. 79, italics in original). Terminology aside, it would have been better to at least have made the distinction between (1) negative affect associated with the *presence* of a fearful situation and (2) negative affect associated with the *absence* of a reward. The former might be dubbed "communal anxiety" and the latter "agentic anxiety," and we would also wish to preserve Sullivan's notion that the two are related in complex ways. As we will discuss in the next section, such a distinction might clarify the relation between anxiety and Sullivan's concepts of *security* and *self-esteem,* respectively.

Roy Baumeister's (1990) exclusion theory of anxiety is a recent and, in fact, postmodern clarification of both the nature and function of anxiety in interpersonal relationships. According to this theory, "anxiety operates as an alarm signal that alerts the individual to the danger of social exclusion" (p. 266). Because the theory "holds that a wide number and variety of groups and relationships hold the potential for causing anxiety by excluding the individual" (p. 263), it departs from the almost-exclusive emphasis given to the mother–infant relationship by psychodynamic theorists (Bowlby, 1969, 1973; Sullivan, 1953a), viewing that relationship as "an especially vivid and important instance of the more general pattern of social exclusion" (p. 263).

In enumerating three general reasons why individuals are excluded from groups, Baumeister distinguished (1) being socially unattractive and acting in ways that alienate others ("unattractive"); (2) failing to make adequate contributions to the success or survival of a group ("incompetent"); and (3) breaking the norms and rules of a group ("immoral"). Baumeister characterized the negative affects associated with each of these exclusion situations as "social anxiety," "performance anxiety," and "guilt," respectively (p. 267). The latter distinctions would seem to parallel rather closely those made by Freud (1933/1964) among neurotic, realistic, and moral anxiety.

From the developmental perspective of Sullivan, it would appear that all three forms of anxiety stem necessarily from the principle of communal existence and are in that sense compatible with Baumeister's general principle of social exclusion. When conjoined with the Foas' developmental theory of social exchange, it would also appear that in older children and adults, the three exclusion situations distinguished by Baumeister also differ in the social resources that are perceived to be at risk. Thus, "social anxiety" is experienced primarily in response to possible loss of love, "performance anxiety" is experienced primarily in response to possible loss of status, and "guilt" is experienced in response to possible loss of both love and status.

From the dyadic–interactional perspective, it is useful to view the negative affect associated with interpersonal situations involving possible loss of love as "communal anxiety" and the negative affect associated with possible loss of status as "agentic anxiety." More important, we conceive of these two dimensions of situations as being orthogonal to one another and would anticipate that most anxiety arousing situations would represent a *mixture* or blend of the two dimensions. We would also anticipate that a circumplex would be the model of choice for scaling situations with reference to their potential for arousing communal and agentic anxiety.

The "unattractive" and "incompetent" grounds for social exclusion described by Baumeister would appear to be reasonably prototypical representations of situations giving rise to communal and agentic anxiety, respectively. The characterization of Baumeister's "immoral" grounds for social exclusion as involving a mixture of communal and agentic apprehensions is not without precedent. For example, Hartmann and Lowenstein (1964) postulated two carrot-and-stick regulatory substructures of the superego system: the ego-ideal (source of experience of pride associated with acting in accord with internalized standards) and the conscience (source of moral anxiety associated with failure to live up to internalized standards). Breaking (internalized) rules and norms of a group may result in loss of both status and love.

Although different reasons for possible exclusion are likely to elicit different blends of agentic and communal anxiety, there are also likely to be differences among individuals in their susceptibility to different sources of anxiety. Highly communal individuals would not wish to alienate others and would probably be sufficiently socialized to avoid breaking rules, although they might experience less "pride" than most for their good behavior. Highly agentic individuals, on the other hand, would want to be recognized for outstanding contributions to the success and survival of their group, but would be less concerned with alienation from others and with conformance to group norms.

Satisfaction, Security, and Self-Esteem

Although Sullivan did not attempt a detailed taxonomy of human motives, his concept of need tensions would seem to apply to a variety of states of disequilibrium created by deficits, the restoration of which results in a state of *satisfaction*. These "gross human motivations" range from biological needs of hunger, thirst, and lust to more psychogenic needs for contact, intimacy, and tenderness. What they have in common are corresponding patterns of overt or covert activity that may "achieve, approach, compromise, or suppress action towards the objective" (Sullivan, 1948, p. 4). Simply put, one can do something about them, and the directionality they impart to behavior is readily understandable.

"The tension called anxiety primarily appertains to the infant's . . . communal existence with a *personal* environment. . . . I distinguish this tension from the sundry tensions already called needs by saying that the relaxation of the tension of anxiety . . . is the experience, not of satisfaction, but of interpersonal *security*" (Sullivan, 1953a, p. 42, italics in original). Because anxiety lacks specific sources of disequilibration, "there is in "the infant no capacity for action toward the relief of anxiety" (p. 42). In short, one can do nothing about anxiety, and its relation to behavior is not immediately evident.[5] Although the term "security" is not further elaborated here, it would seem, in this context, to suggest a freedom from anxiety about separation (Bowlby, 1973) or exclusion (Baumeister, 1990) from a communal environment.

The term "security" reappears in Sullivan's (1953a) later discussion (in the same work) of the developmental epoch of early adolescence: "by security I mean one's feelings of *self-esteem* and personal worth" (p. 266, italics added). Elsewhere he states, "The observed failure of someone to treat us with the deference which we had expected him to show calls out anxiety" (Sullivan, 1948, p. 11). The ambiguity here is whether what would appear to us to be "communal anxiety" occurs only in infancy and perhaps serves as a precursor to adult "agentic anxiety" or whether both communal and agentic anxiety are the major motivating forces in adult interpersonal behavior.

Contemporary interpersonal theorists clearly favor some form of the "both" interpretation, although they are hard put to find documentation for it in the writings of Sullivan. For example, Swensen (1973) assumes that both motives are present in infancy: "disapproval threatens the infant's self-esteem and security and, thus, produces anxiety. . . . Anything that threatens self-esteem or security produces anxiety" (p. 22). The conjunctions (and, or) are critical here and may be ambiguous, as in the often-employed characterization of Sullivan's position on major motives as being "to avoid anxiety *and* maintain self-esteem." In more recent times, Benjamin (1993) dealt with the problem candidly: "To paraphrase Sullivan loosely, he held that love and power are the fundamental needs and that anxiety is the basic fear" (p. 16).

The principal source for contemporary views of interpersonal motives was most likely Timothy Leary (1957), according to whose close reading of Sullivan, "*Anxiety is interpersonal because it is rooted in the dreaded expectation of derogation and rejection by others (or by oneself)*" (p. 8, italics added). Perhaps we could accept this interpretation as Sullivanian in spirit, "if not in all details."[6] It coincides nicely with the Foas' later formulations regarding the giving (status and love) and taking away (derogation and rejection) of interpersonal resources, and it is compatible with many of Sullivan's more valuable contributions. To simplify matters, let us consider *satisfaction* as being related primarily to the resources of services, goods, money, and information; *security* as being related to communal needs (love); and *self-esteem* as being related to agentic needs (status). Now consider Sullivan's (1953b) succinct and compelling definition of "love": "*When the satisfaction or the security of another person becomes as significant to one as is one's own satisfaction or security, then the state of love exists*" (pp. 42–43, italics in original). In this context, does "security" mean self-esteem, a sense of being loved, or both?

Personality Defined

Personality is the relatively enduring pattern of recurrent interpersonal situations which characterize a human life.
—SULLIVAN (1953b, pp. 110–111)

This is not the usual notion of a "separate" personality existing in the context of a situation, nor is it simply the idea of one person interacting with another. And it is most decidedly not a statistical interaction abstracted from an analysis of person and situation variance. What *is* being conveyed here can only be suggested by considering a few examples of the several components that constitute this rich and tightly packed definition of personality.

"Relatively Enduring"

Sullivan's (1953a) theory of motivation, like that of Freud's, was grounded in metapsychological propositions expressed in the physical language of energy and force. The concept of dynamism was defined as: *"the relatively enduring pattern of energy transformations which recurrently characterize the organism in its duration as a living organism"* (p. 103, italics in original). As applied to interpersonal relationships, the function of tensions, associated with needs, is to *sustain* overt actions directed toward "bringing about the appearance, approach, and cooperation of [an appropriate other] in connection with the satisfaction of a need" (p. 92).

"Pattern"

Sullivan's (1953a) definition of *pattern* as *"the envelope of insignificant particular differences"* (p. 104, italics in original), although formidable at first encounter, is well worth considering. This would appear to be mainly a technical point concerning the psychophysics of pattern recognition that is nonetheless remarkable, considering the time at which it was suggested. The definition refers to the point or "limit" at which detectable variations in a pattern depart significantly enough from a standard configuration (prototype?) to change the judged category membership of the observed pattern. Thus, as Sullivan notes, although a fruit remains an "orange" under insignificant variations in size, shape, and skin texture, significant variations in these or other characteristics lead us to assign the fruit to some other botanical category (e.g., tangerine).

The slides that Sullivan (1948) used to illustrate a later lecture on his concept of pattern bear an almost eerie resemblance to the principal model under consideration in the present chapter[7]:

> Let me now take the risk of hopelessly misleading many of you by using a perhaps ill-conceived visual aid to indicate how the "purely personal" can actually be very really the interpersonal.

In Fig. [4.2], I show a way of depicting "a personality," the hypothetical entity which we posit to account for interpersonal fields. . . . Each of these sectors in itself indicates a major motivational system. Please do not think that there are but six major motivational systems; it is convenient to draw six sectors. (p. 6)

In Fig. [4.3] we are no longer concerned with the representation of a hypothetical personality but with depicting an instance of an interpersonal situation, the sort of thing that can be studied by a psychiatrist. . . . You will note that the uppermost line representing a field force is cross-hatched. This is intended to represent force which tends to keep these two people from growing intimate, what might be called disjunctive force. . . . Below that are shown two dotted lines of force which represent conjunctive forces. (p. 7)

This striking example of Sullivan's "foresight" with respect to contemporary interpersonal circumplex models is made even more remarkable by its illumination of what has been, apparently, a lack of "hindsight" with respect to this aspect of Sullivan's work on the part of more recent investigators in the field.

"Of Recurrent Interpersonal Situations"

Psychiatry (as Sullivan, 1953b, conceived it) "seeks to study the biologically and culturally conditioned, but *sui generis* (one of a kind), interpersonal processes occurring in the interpersonal situations in which the observant psychiatrist does his work" (p. 20). In particular, the psychiatrist focuses on complementary needs inferred from reciprocal patterns of activity on the respective parts of the patient and the psychiatrist. Such reciprocal patterns result in future reintegration (*recurrence*) of a particular interpersonal situation (Sullivan, 1954). This "theorem of reciprocal emotion" was more complex in its original presentation by Sullivan than in its subsequent application to the laboratory investigation of dyadic interactions (e.g., Orford, 1986). A single example presented by Sullivan (1954) must suffice.

A patient with a diminished sense of self-esteem may have developed the defensive pattern of discounting, disbelieving, or converting to its opposite all attempts by significant others to praise the patient directly. Should this defensive pattern occur in interviews with a psychiatrist, the need of the psychiatrist to reassure would not be complementary to the patient's need to avoid, alleviate, or escape

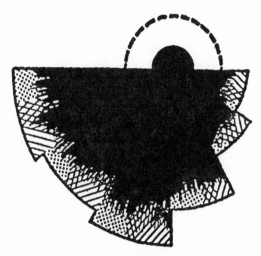

FIGURE 4.2. Sullivan's depiction of the major motivational systems of personality as sectors of a circle. From Sullivan (1948, p. 6). Copyright 1948 by the William Alanson White Psychiatric Foundation. Reprinted by permission.

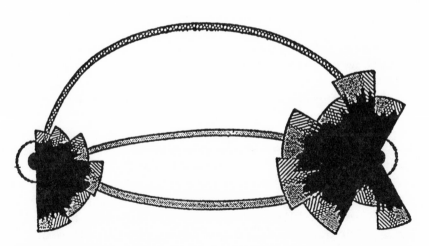

FIGURE 4.3. Sullivan's depiction of a dyadic interpersonal situation involving disjunctive and conjunctive field forces. From Sullivan (1948, p. 7). Copyright 1948 by the William Alanson White Psychiatric Foundation. Reprinted by permission.

from anxiety over self-esteem, and both participants might realize that the situation is disintegrating: "Most psychiatrists have had this unpleasant retrospective realization that they have said, or permitted the patient to say without rejoinder, something which is seriously discouraging. . . . In some instances, the patient is so far ahead of the psychiatrist that he soon realizes that things are not going to work" (p. 126). Under these circumstances, the astute psychiatrist might recognize that "reassuring by implication" is the pattern of activity that is reciprocal to the patient's pattern of discounting and disbelieving. Reassuring by implication would involve "saying something which would have very little to do with the other person's self-esteem, but would, on further elaboration, be seen to imply a favorable view or hopeful outlook" (p. 129). Such a pattern would foster further recurrence "on the basis of either witting or unnoted anticipation of improvement of one's self-esteem in or by the relationship" (p. 130).

Sullivan provided detailed descriptions of the complex processes whereby interpersonal situations are (1) *resolved* and integrated by complementary needs and reciprocal patterns of activity and, hence, likely to recur; (2) *continued* with tension and exploration of alternative avenues to satisfactory resolution; or (3) *frustrated*, leading to possible disintegration and nonrecurrence of the situation. Although these processes were formulated within the context of the psychiatric interview (Sullivan, 1954, Chap. 6), they were meant to apply *generally*: "The interpersonal processes making up the interview follow the general pattern of all interpersonal processes" (p. 132). Thus, the psychiatric interview would seem to provide a unique microcosm of transactions in which interpersonal processes can be minutely observed and even manipulated by interventions of the interviewer.

A possible limit on the generalizability of observations made within the psychiatric interview is the comparatively low status and prestige associated with the patient's role: "By cultural definition, the patient is the client of an expert, and therefore is inferior in significant respects" (p. 131), and with respect to the psychiatrist, "those who come to him must be relatively insecure" (p. 12). In virtually all of the case-history material presented by Sullivan (1954), anxiety in both interviewer and interviewee, is interpreted with reference to *self-esteem* ("security" in Sullivan's terms). This may reflect in part the fact that therapist–patient transactions occur in the context of primarily *agentic situations* (see Moscowitz, 1994). The extent to which anxiety occurs with reference to possible loss of love ("security" in our usage) in other, primarily *communal situations* (e.g., romantic partners) is an open question.

"Which Characterize a Human Life"

Sullivan (1956) was impressed with the extent to which habitual patterns of interpersonal transactions may be said to characterize a human life, despite variations in situational demands. For example, when a stranger defines an uncharacteristic role for us, "we carry on quite well in living up to that role for a while; but as the impression of strangeness wears off, as we begin to pick up some notions about the other fellow, we also begin to be somewhat worn out with the unfamiliar restraints that we are exercising on ourselves, and more and more of our habitual personality or habitual type of interpersonal relation comes into play" (p. 200).

As stated earlier, Sullivan sought to study interpersonal processes that he viewed as "one-of-a-kind," that is, singularly characteristic of the individual studied. Consequently, he was concerned about forcing patients into Kraepelinian diagnostic categories that failed to capture their unique patterns of interpersonal transactions. In this context, he advoctated "factual diagnosis" rather than "formal diagnosis" (Sullivan, 1956, p. 193). His approach to psychiatric diagnosis was motivated more by an interest in *what can be done* for a patient than by an interest in labeling an illness. This approach involved two frames of reference. "The first of these is the viewing of each case in terms of the outstanding *difficulties in living,* the liabilities, as against the degree of ability demonstrated to meet complex situations, the assets" (p. 195, emphasis added). The second frame of reference aims to determine the specific "tools and facilities" available to the psychotherapist and the likely motivation of the patient for taking advantage of such facilities.

Sullivan's emphasis on difficulties in living reflected his interest in the *adaptive* consequences of characteristic interpersonal patterns. In this context, he recognized that there are "recurrent eccentricities in interpersonal relations" (Sullivan, 1954, p. 195) that are associated with diagnostic categories such as hysteria, obsessionalism, manic–depressive psychosis, and schizophrenia (Sullivan, 1956, Part II). Nevertheless, he emphasized that *all* of these diagnostic patterns "may also appear in any of us." Such patterns become dysfunctional when they are applied inappropriately or inflexibly. "Behavior that might be useful for something or other is used by these people to meet problems for which it is singularly ineffective, or . . . [these] people do something that every one of us does at some time during the day, but they do it almost all the time, and thereby seem very eccentric indeed" (Sullivan, 1954, p. 195). This quantitative rather than qualitative difference between normal and disordered personalities underlies Sullivan's (1953a) observation that "*everyone is much more simply human than otherwise*" (p. 32, italics in original).

Measurement of Interpersonal Behavior

Let me say that insofar as you are interested in your unique individuality, in contradistinction to the interpersonal activities that you or someone else can observe, to that extent you are interested in the really private mode in which you live—in which I have no interest whatever.
                                                            —SULLIVAN (1953a, p. 19)

Units of Observation

It follows from Sullivan's definition of personality that the "individual" cannot be considered apart from the interpersonal situation in which he or she is engaged. Moreover, in contrast to the predominant Freudian view of his time, Sullivan emphasized the observation of what persons actually *do* to one another, rather than speculating upon what intrapsychic conflicts they might "have." What persons do in social situations can be described by a verb (help), the effect of their actions upon another can be described by an adjective (helpful), and the social role that they play can sometimes be described by a noun (helper). Because the basic unit of observation is an interpersonal situation rather than an "individual" act, the implications of a given action for *both* actor and recipient must be specified.

In the act of *helping*, an actor may grant both love and status to the other. Giving love to another is associated with giving love to self; granting status to another reduces (however slightly) one's own status. Hence, the "helper" defines the *interpersonal situation* as:

Self [status (−1); love (+1)] and *Other* [love (+1); status (+1)]

From the theorem of reciprocal emotion, one might anticipate that the helped-other would experience an increase in both self-esteem and security, and view the helper as one who gives love and loses status. Hence, the "helped-other" defines the *interpersonal situation* as:

Self [status (+1); love (+1)] and *Other* [love (+1); status (−1)]

The notation we are using here is an adaptation of Foa's (1965) facet analysis of interpersonal variables that provides a "systematic definition of the set of variables in terms of more basic sets, the facets, [and] leads to the prediction of the empirical interrelationships among the variables" (p. 262). Briefly, from his cognitive-developmental theory of personality, Foa reasoned that interpersonal variables could be decomposed into three facets: (a) *object* (self and other), (b) *resource* (love and status), and (c) *directionality* [giving (+1) and taking away (−1)]. The facet composition of the interpersonal variables we have employed in our own research is given in Table 4.4a. The verbal labels we have assigned to these variables are (PA) assured–dominant, (BC) arrogant–calculating, (DE) cold-hearted, (FG) aloof–introverted, (HI) unassured–submissive, (JK) unassuming–ingenuous, (LM) warm–agreeable, and (NO) gregarious–extraverted.

From the seventh row of Table 4.4a, it can be seen that the helping act we have been discussing would be coded as a warm–agreeable variable (LM), in which the actor defined the interpersonal situation as one in which love, but not status, was granted to self while both love and status were granted to the helped-other. More substantively, this variable has been described as the providing of "material or emotional benefits to others who are in trouble, who need help, who are ill, or who are otherwise in need of care and support" (Wiggins, 1995, p. 26).

Interpersonal variables of this kind may be conceptualized and measured on several *levels* ranging from "microanalytic behavioral sequences as when the behavior of person A is identified as a particular response and a particular stimulus in an ongoing transaction cycle with person B . . . to macroanalytic analyses of ongoing relationships emphasizing enduring patterns of behavior" (Pincus, 1994, p. 115). Our helping example was on the microanalytic level in which A's warm–agreeable (LM) response was a stimulus for B's assured–dominant (PA) reaction (see Table 4.4a). Response-by-response analyses on this level provide the basic data for the investigation of such topics as the theorem of reciprocal emotion and "complementarity" in interpersonal transactions. Macroanalytic analyses

TABLE 4.4. Derivation of the Interpersonal Circumplex

a. Facet composition of interpersonal variables

	Self		Other	
	Status	Love	Love	Status
PA	+1	+1	+1	−1
BC	+1	+1	−1	−1
DE	+1	−1	−1	−1
FG	−1	−1	−1	−1
HI	−1	−1	−1	+1
JK	−1	−1	+1	+1
LM	−1	+1	+1	+1
NO	+1	+1	+1	+1

b. Sums of cross-products (ΣXY)

	PA	BC	DE	FG	HI
PA	4				
BC	2	4			
DE	0	2	4		
FG	−2	0	2	4	
HI	−4	−2	0	2	4
JK	−2	−4	−2	0	2
LM	0	−2	−4	−2	0
NO	2	0	−2	−4	−2

c. Correlation matrix ($\Sigma XY/N$)

	PA	BC	DE	FG	HI
PA	1.00				
BC	.50	1.00			
DE	.00	.50	1.00		
FG	−.50	.00	.50	1.00	
HI	−1.00	−.50	.00	.50	1.00
JK	−.50	−1.00	−.50	.00	.50
LM	.00	−.50	−1.00	−.50	.00
NO	.50	.00	−.50	−1.00	−.50

d. Rotated factor matrix

	I	II	h^2
PA	.92	.00	.85
BC	.65	−.65	.85
DE	.00	−.92	.85
FG	−.65	−.65	.85
HI	−.92	.00	.85
JK	−.65	.65	.85
LM	.00	.92	.85
NO	.65	.65	.85
% Var.	42.5%	42.5%	85%

of patterns of interpersonal behavior that endure over time and situations are concerned with *interpersonal traits* that, in differing configurations, reflect characteristic interpersonal styles or modes of adaptation.

The Structure of Interpersonal Behavior

The facet composition of interpersonal variables in Table 4.4a serves both to define the variables and to generate predictions as to their interrelations. From the rows of Table 4.4a, it can be seen that the facet composition of each variable differs from its preceding variable by only one element. The BC variable (arrogant–calculating) differs from its preceding PA variable (assured–dominant) in not granting love to the other; the DE variable (cold-hearted) differs from its preceding BC variable in not granting love to self, and so on. Note also that the last variable (NO) differs from the first variable (PA) by only one element; the assured–dominant variable does not grant status to the other. To the extent that this hypothesized pattern of facets for the set of eight interpersonal variables is correct, the relations among indicants of the eight variables will be *circular*. This may be illustrated with some simple calculations.

The relation between any two variables in Table 4.4a may be estimated by summing the cross-products of their respective row elements. Thus, the relation between PA and BC is determined by:

$$(+1 * +1) + (+1 * +1) + (+1 * -1) + (-1 * -1) = 2$$

The sums of the cross-products for all combinations of the eight variables are presented in Table 4.4b. The sum of the cross-products of any variable with itself is 4, and these numbers appear in the main diagonal. Dividing the elements in Table 4.4b by the number of "observations" (4) yields the more familiar matrix of Table 4.4c, which some may recognize as a *circulant* correlation matrix (Guttman, 1954). Extracting and rotating two principal components from the matrix in Table 4.4c yields the factor matrix presented in Table 4.4d.

Table 4.4 is meant to demonstrate that if the *hypothesized* facet composition of variables in Table 4.4a is in fact true, then the structural relations among variables will form a circulant matrix (Table 4.4c), the underlying component structure of which necessarily forms a circumplex. Several restrictions on inference in this situation must be immediately noted. First of all, even granting that love and status are the social resources exchanged, their assigned facet values across variables in Table 4.4a are not unique. Any arrangement of facet values in which adjacent variables (and the first and last variables) differ by one element will yield a circulant matrix. Thus, Table 4.4a provides a set of hypotheses whose empirical validation requires extensive work. To take a single example: D. M. Buss's (1991a) finding that husbands and wives of dominant (PA) spouses complained that their spouses were condescending (e.g., "He or she treated me like I was stupid or inferior") may be considered a confirmation of the denial of status to other in the first row of Table 4.4a. Other forms of evidence considered relevant to the validation of facet composition matrices are discussed by Wiggins (1982, pp. 213–217).

A great deal of both conceptual and empirical effort has been expended in evaluating the extent to which interpersonal variables conform to the type of structure illustrated in Table 4.4d. A broader theoretical issue here is whether such structural characteristics are "discovered" or "imposed" upon scales measuring interpersonal variables (Loevinger, 1957, pp. 661–676). In accord with strategies suggested by Loevinger, our preliminary studies of the universe of content of interpersonal behavior were conducted within a context of discovery that provided a theoretical basis for the item-selection procedures we later employed in developing optimal scale sets to map this universe. Figure 4.4 presents the *empirical* circumplex structure of the Interpersonal Adjective Scales (IAS; Wiggins, 1995), obtained in a sample of college students. With respect to several indices of "goodness of fit" of a circumplex, this solution conforms well to both conceptual and empirical criteria (see Wiggins, 1995, pp. 46–48). Such a result is of the utmost importance, because the measurement operations to be described next are predicated on the assumption that interpersonal measuring instruments, such as IAS, meet stringent geometric and substantive criteria.

Interpersonal Space

Universe of Content

The two coordinates of the circular plane illustrated in Figure 4.4 provide a conceptual definition of the universe of content of interpersonal behavior in terms of the metaconcepts of agency and communion. On a more concrete level, these coordinates are rotational variants of the first two factors of the five-factor model that we describe as dominance and nurturance. In principle, any dyadic interaction that has social (status) and emotional (love) implications for both participants (self and other) may be classified within this space. Consider the IAS gregarious–extraverted scale (NO), for example. The angular location of this scale is 45°, which is the midpoint of the "NO sector" that ranges from 22° to 67°. Items, scales, or persons falling at this location are considered to be prototypically

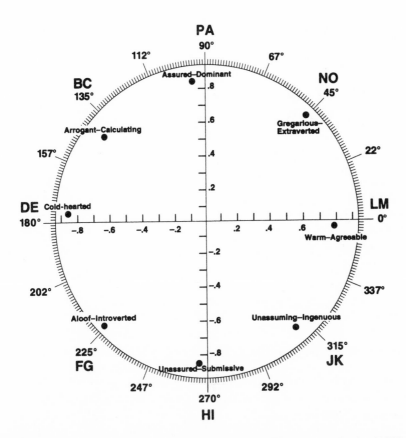

FIGURE 4.4. Circumplex structure of IAS scales (*N* = 2,988). From Wiggins (1995, p. 4). Adapted and reproduced by special permission of the Publisher, Psychological Assessment Resources, Inc., Odessa, FL 33556, from the Interpersonal Adjective Scales–Revised by Jerry S. Wiggins, Ph.D. Copyright 1995 by PAR, Inc. Further reproduction is prohibited without permission from PAR, Inc.

gregarious–extraverted, an equal "blend" of the dominance and nurturance coordinates. Items, scales, or persons falling toward 67° will be "stronger"; those falling toward 22° will be "warmer." Note also that the distance of the IAS gregarious–extraverted scale from the center of the circle is .88 (out of a possible 1.00). We refer to this trigonometric value as "vector length," and in the present example would interpret it as an index of how well the variance of the IAS gregarious–extraverted scale is captured by the *interpersonal* coordinates of this space, a quality Gurtman (1991) has dubbed "interpersonalness." Scales with near-zero vector lengths are, by definition, *not* interpersonal in content. Such scales are likely to have loadings on one or more of the three remaining dimensions of the five-factor model; analytic procedures for determining this are available (Hofstee et al., 1992).

Microanalytic Measurement

When interpersonal space is interpreted on the microanalytic level, it provides a framework for the systematic observation of ongoing interpersonal transactions. The pioneering studies of the Kaiser Foundation Group (Freedman, Leary, Ossorio, & Coffey, 1951) were based on ordinary language descriptions of interpersonal transactions in small groups, from which "the circle emerged" (LaForge, 1977, p. 8). Quite independently, Bales (1950) developed a highly similar coding system for describing social interactions in small groups. Notable recent microanalytic investigations of interpersonal space include the detailed analysis of prototypcial acts by D. M. Buss and Craik (1983) and the precise mapping of nonverbal behaviors within interpersonal space by Gifford (1991).

Macroanalytic Measurement

When interpersonal space is interpreted on the macroanalytic level, it provides a framework for the systematic investigation of enduring patterns of interpersonal behavior. In this context, Leary (1956) was among the first to emphasize the methodological utility of interpersonal space in the study of individuals, dyads, and groups, and to apply these methods to the clinical assessment of patients, married couples, and families. The literature of interpersonal traits is now so extensive that is can only be selectively illustrated in the material that follows.

Interpersonal Profiles

The coordinates of interpersonal space may be employed to characterize the dispositional tendencies of individuals with reference to profiles of variables of the kind illustrated in Figure 4.5. Although the procedures for "profile analysis" of interpersonal dispositions are in some ways similar to those employed for other sets of psychometric measures, they differ in the extent to which the order and structure of the constituent variables are systematically patterned within a defined and fully sampled universe of content. As Gurtman and Balakrishnan (1994) put it,

> In a sense, much of conventional profile patterning is the product of happenstance—as scales often have no natural order, any particular sequencing of scores is simply a device of tradition. Thus, classic MMPI/MMPI-2 profile types, such as the "conversion V" and "paranoid valley," are partly artifact: they might have assumed different forms (and hence different monikers) had circumstances produced some other linear arrangement of MMPI scales. (p. 10)

The Kaiser Foundation Group (LaForge, Leary, Naboisek, Coffey, & Freedman, 1954) was the first to exploit the geometric properties of a circle for representing interpersonal tendencies by a profile, and the clinical–diagnostic utility of such representations was later demonstrated convincingly by Leary (1957). The circular profile of variables shown in Figure 4.5 may be used to illustrate the unique features of this approach. First, the overall shape of the profile has a *characteristic configuration* of interpersonal tendencies that we call an "interpersonal spaceship," in this instance one traveling due west.[8] The highest elevation occurs on the defining octant (DE), followed by adjacent octants (BC and FG), and diminishing to the highly truncated opposite octant (LM). The "directionality" of this profile may be determined more precisely by calculating the mean or average of the eight vectors with reference to the polar coordinates of angle and vector length (distance from the center of the circle). In this profile, the mean angular direction is 178 and the vector length is 71 (T-score units with $\bar{X} = 50$ and $SD = 10$).

The angular direction of the profile in Figure 4.5 falls near the midpoint of the cold-hearted octant and would result in a "diagnosis" of the individual producing this profile as a "DE Type." Profiles falling closer to the BC boundary of this type (e.g., 158) would be "stronger" in the expression of anger, and profiles falling closer to the FG boundary (e.g., 200) would be "weaker" (i.e., more withdrawn). But the present profile is near the midpoint of DE and hence would be considered as *prototypical* of this category. This conceptualization of circumplex categories as fuzzy sets with continuous (as opposed to discrete) class membership (Wiggins, 1980) retains some of the advantages of both categorical and dimensional approaches to typological diagnosis (Widiger & Frances, 1994).

When a person is assigned to the cold-hearted category, it is anticipated that he or she will often behave in ways that emphasize autonomy and freedom from social conventions, and that he or she

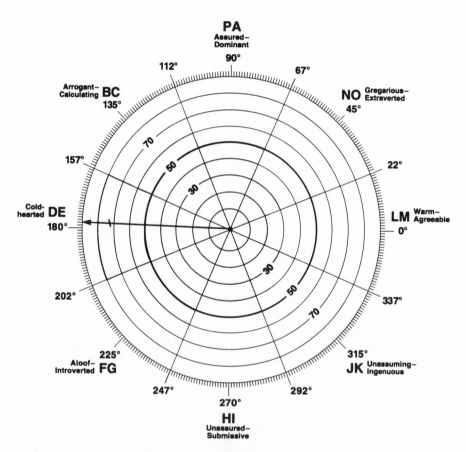

FIGURE 4.5. Illustrative IAS profile of a cold-hearted (DE) type. From Wiggins (1995, p. 21). Adapted and reproduced by special permission of the Publisher, Psychological Assessment Resources, Inc., Odessa, FL 33556, from the Interpersonal Adjective Scales—Revised by Jerry S. Wiggins, Ph.D. Copyright 1995 by PAR, Inc. Further reproduction is prohibited without permission from PAR, Inc.

will tend *not* to be warm, cooperative, or nurturant when such behaviors would be appropriate (Wiggins, 1995, p. 24). On the basis of the "characteristic configuration" notion discussed earlier, it is *also* anticipated that a cold-hearted person (DE) will, somewhat less frequently, behave in an arrogant–calculating manner (BC) and that the person will seldom (if ever) behave in a warm–agreeable way (LM), and so forth. How often and with what intensity this characteristic pattern will be manifest is assumed to be related to the vector length value of the profile. In the present example, this value (71) is two standard deviations above average, leading to the expectation that this definitely "noncommunal" style will be painfully evident to others. An additional basis for this prediction is the angular location of this profile (178°), which suggests a high degree of prototypicality. A more empirically based measure of prototypicality can be obtained by determining the "fit" of the present profile to established norms for members of the DE category, using the computational procedures described by Gurtman (1994).

Even this fragmentary example of interpersonal profile interpretation makes clear that there are strong geometric and substantive assumptions involved when assessment instruments are used to classify persons into typological categories defined by the coordinates of interpersonal space. A number of these assumptions have been subjected to empirical test and the results have been, for the most part, highly encouraging (e.g., Wiggins et al., 1989). The congruence between theory and data in interpersonal assessment is, at times, so close that it is unclear whether the interpretive enterprise is theoretically or empirically "driven," a process we have described as "circular reasoning." Criteria for an ultimate model of personality structure have ranged from "adequate" (Norman, 1963) to "compelling" (Goldberg, 1982). Although much work remains to be done within the interpersonal domain, our own expectations for eventually understanding this domain are closer to the Pollyannaish end of the scale just implied.

Interpersonal Contexts

Although the realm of interpersonal behavior is a domain of individual differences that may be distinguished from other domains (e.g., the remaining three factors of the FFM), there are different contexts of measurement *within* the interpersonal domain whose conceptual relations to one another are less easy to articulate. Historically, this problem first arose in the Freedman et al. (1951) original distinction among three "levels" of measurement in the interpersonal system (public, conscious, and private), to which Leary (1957) added the levels of unexpressed and values. LaForge (1963) argued that different *methods* of measurement were being distinguished rather than different "levels," and Wiggins (1965) noted that "the standards whereby one would evaluate the extent to which the *same* variables are involved at *different* levels are not specified so that one is uncertain as to whether convergent or discriminant validation would be assessed in cross-level correlations" (p. 453, italics in original).

The question raised 30 years ago (Wiggins, 1965) has not been completely answered, but instead has assumed a new and arguably more productive form. The conceptual units of observation and the structure of interpersonal space are now sufficiently "standard" that it is possible to examine some of the *contexts* in which the model might be fruitfully employed in the absence of a grand scheme for relating these contexts to one another. The term "context" is used here primarily because it carries less surplus meaning than do "levels" or "methods." Four examples will have to suffice as illustrations of different contexts of measurement within the interpersonal domain.

Interpersonal Dispositions

It seems appropriate that the original context in which interpersonal behavior was explored was that of interpersonal *traits*: "human tendencies (pronenesses, proclivities, propensities, dispositions, inclinations) to act or not to act in certain ways on certain occasions" (Wiggins, in press). The enduring centrality of the trait concept in personality psychology is evident in both the recent empirical literature of that field (Wiggins & Pincus, 1992) and in the multiple theoretical perspectives presented in this volume. Our own early work (Wiggins, 1979) approached traits from a lexical perspective (Saucier & Goldberg, Chapter 2, this volume) within which we made a priori distinctions among such trait categories as *interpersonal* (e.g., "dominant," "nurturant"), *character* (e.g., "scrupulous"), *temperament* (e.g., "nervous"), and *mental predicates* (e.g., "philosophical"). The painstaking work of earlier personality lexicologists (e.g., Norman, 1967) provided us with an exceptionally broad and inclusive definition of the universe of content of interpersonal traits. The Interpersonal Adjective Scales (IAS; Wiggins, 1995) were derived within this framework.

Interpersonal Problems

Interpersonal dispositions do not always operate in ways that are adaptive. Difficulties in living may result when traits are expressed rigidly or excessively, or when they are *not* expressed in situations in which they would be clearly adaptive. In this context, the focus is on the *problematic* nature of dispositions (for self and/or others), rather than on the relative frequency of occurrence of dispositions. "An individual having strong interpersonal dispositions will not *necessarily* manifest interpersonal problems; however, individuals who do manifest interpersonal problems would be likely to have the corresponding dispositions underlying such problems" (Pincus & Wiggins, 1990, p. 344).

Horowitz (1979) defined the universe of content of interpersonal problems with reference to the problems in living expressed by psychiatric outpatients in the course of videotaped intake interviews. Two observers viewed the videotaped interviews and recorded problem statements expressing excesses (e.g., "I try to please other people too much") and inhibitions (e.g., "It's hard for me to trust other people"). Problem statements that were not interpersonal in nature ("I have trouble falling asleep at night") were excluded from the item pool. Meaning–similarity ratings of this item pool were subjected to multidimensional scaling procedures that yielded two dimensions strongly suggestive of interpersonal space. The resultant Inventory of Interpersonal Problems (IIP; Horowitz, Rosenberg, Baer, Ureno, & Villasenor, 1988) presents these items in a self-report format in which "How much have you been distressed by this problem?" is rated on a five-place scale for each item.

Alden, Wiggins, and Pincus (1990) developed a circumplex version (IIP-C) of the Inventory of Interpersonal Problems, consisting of eight octant scales that mark the appropriate sectors of interpersonal space, for example, (PA) domineering, (BC) vindictive, (DE) cold, and so on. The circumplex structure of IIP-C is remarkably robust (e.g., Soldz, Budman, Demby, & Merry, 1993) and the instrument has proven useful in both research (e.g., Gurtman, 1992b) and clinical (e.g., Pincus & Wiggins, 1992) settings. It is also important to note that the items of IIP-C are distributed continuously around the circumplex (Wiggins, 1991b), thereby establishing that Horowitz's (1979) original sampling of the universe of content was successful. Although developed independently of IAS, the circumplex scales of IIP-C exhibit strong structural convergences with that instrument within a common interpersonal space (Alden et al., 1990, pp. 532–533). The still unanswered question of how the variables from the two contexts "differ" from one another would seem to require further explorations of their discriminant validities.

Impact Messages

The Impact Message Inventory (IMI; Kiesler, 1987) was developed in a context that differed radically from those of the instruments discussed thus far. The concept of "impact message" is central to Kiesler's (1979, 1982, 1983, 1988) theory of interpersonal communication in psychotherapy. When you (the reader) interact with an assured–dominant partner, you may, upon introspection, come to realize that your partner evokes certain *feelings* in you ("bossed around"), certain action *tendencies* ("I want to tell him to give someone else a chance to make a decision"), and certain *perceptions of an evoking message* ("He thinks he's always in control of things"). These covert "impacts" that your partner has upon you are conceptually distinct from your own interpersonal dispositions and from your partner's interpersonal dispositions; they reflect the way your partner affects you (and probably others), and your partner may or may not be aware of how he or she "comes across" in social transactions. Nevertheless, these subtle communications are well captured by interpersonal space.

In the development of the IMI, Kiesler (1987) first constructed 15 interpersonal vignettes, in paragraph form, to typify the overt interpersonal behaviors suggested by items from the 15 categories of Lorr and NcNair's (1967) Interpersonal Behavior Inventory. These descriptions of interpersonal styles were next presented to members of Kiesler's research team with instructions "to imagine themselves in the company of each of the persons described and to record their free-response covert reactions using the sentence stem, *He makes me feel . . .* " (p. 5). The 784 items, thus generated, defined the universe of content of impact messages. The majority of these items were reliably classified into the three subcategories of feelings, action tendencies, and perceived evoking messages, described earlier. Fifteen IMI scales were then constructed by procedures that maximized the alignment of subsets of impact items with their corresponding interpersonal behavior categories on the Lorr–McNair circumplex. We constructed an eight-scale "octant version" of the IMI using the same analytic methods we had employed in the development of the IAS and IIP-C. Kiesler and Schmidt (1991) have scored this octant version within their own varied groups of subjects and, although not as robust as the IAS and IIP-C, the octant version of the IMI provides an acceptable circumplex solution that clearly spans interpersonal space (Kiesler & Schmidt, 1991). The utility of the original version of the IMI has been most convincingly demonstrated in research on personality, psychotherapy, and health psychology (Kiesler, 1987). The structural convergence of the IMI octant scales with corresponding IAS scales (Kiesler & Schmidt, 1991, p. 39) may, at the least, be considered another demonstration of the generalizability of dispositional space across interpersonal contexts.

Psychiatric Diagnoses

From the inception of the interpersonal system (e.g., Leary, 1957) to its most recent formulations (e.g., Benjamin, 1993), it has been suggested that the relations among formal categories of psychiatric diagnosis (e.g., "schizoid personality") may be captured by interpersonal space (see Wiggins, 1982). Schaefer and Plutchik (1966), for example, provided evidence that trait terms, emotion terms, and ratings of diagnostic labels share a common interpersonal space. A resurgence of interest in this topic occurred when the third edition of the *Diagnostic and Statistical Manual of Mental Disorders* (DSM-III; American Psychiatric Association, 1980) provided an axis of personality disorders defined *by personality traits* that are inflexible and maladaptive. The substantive similarity of some of the DSM-III categories of personality disorder to the octants of the Interpersonal Circle led to definite, although differing, expectations for their placement within that circle (Kiesler, 1986; Widiger & Kelso, 1983; Wiggins, 1982).

Wiggins (1987) reported preliminary findings suggesting that certain of the personality disorders of DSM-III were well captured by dimensions of the IAS and the NEO-PI, and concluded that "a full understanding of their personological implications can only be achieved within the context of the Big Five dimensions of personality" (p. 10). This conclusion was strongly supported by subsequent work (see Costa & Widiger, 1994). More extensive studies later established that 6 of the 11 categories of personality disorder were well captured by both the dispositional space of the IAS (Wiggins & Pincus, 1989) and the problems space of the IIP (Pincus & Wiggins, 1990). The generalizability of the findings with respect to interpersonal problems was considerably enhanced by a study conducted by Soldz et al. (1993) within a carefully selected sample of psychiatric outpatients who were diagnosed as personality disorders by a structured clinical interview (Loranger, 1988) and were administered the IIP-C and the Millon Clinical Multiaxial Inventory (Millon, 1987).

Societal Perspectives on the Five-Factor Model

In many respects, our view of the FFM is conceptually similar to that held by Robert Hogan (1983; Chapter 5, this volume). Hogan assigns a conceptual priority to two "biologically mandated" human tendencies to meet the societal challenges of "getting ahead" (status hierarchy) and "getting along" (group living). In addition to their similarities to the metaconcepts of agency and communion, these two coordinates are used by Hogan to classify *types* of social/vocational roles through which societal needs are fulfilled, using Holland's (1985a) Vocational Preference Inventory, an inventory that has clear circumplex properties (Tracey & Rounds, 1993; Trapnell, 1989). In this context, Hogan views the dimensions of the FFM as dimensions of *social evaluation* whereby group members judge the competence of individuals for contributing to societal goals.

Our own granting of conceptual priority to the first two factors of the FFM is done so on the grounds of their relative "purity" as lower order indicants of the highly abstract notions of agency and communion. On this view, the remaining dimensions of Conscientiousness, Neuroticism, and Openness/Intellect are viewed as dimensions that either facilitate (desirable) or interfere with (undesirable) the development and maintenance of agentic and communal enterprises within a social group. More radically, we assert that the interpenetration of agentic and communal concerns into the other three factors is so complete that manifestations of both can be identified *within* each of the factors. From the dyadic–interactional perspective, the disagreements in the literature over alternative interpretations of the last three factors of the FFM may be seen as stemming from differing emphases on the *agentic* and *communal* components of each of the factors involved.

Agency, Communion, and Conscientiousness

The ordinary-language meaning of "conscientious" is "controlled by or done according to conscience" (Random House, 1993), which clearly suggests a communal connotation. The apparent consensus that Factor III should be labeled "Conscientiousness" (Botwin & D. M. Buss, 1989; Goldberg, 1990; McCrae & John, 1992; Norman, 1963; Peabody & Goldberg, 1989; Trapnell & Wiggins, 1990) might therefore suggest an agreement on its communal implications, as well. Those who have labeled this factor "Dependability" (Fiske, 1949; Tupes & Christal, 1961/1992), "Conformity" (Hogan, 1983), "Prudence" (Hogan, 1986), and "Constraint" (Tellegen, 1994; Johnson & Ostendorff, 1993) have opted even more clearly for a communal interpretation. And Cattell's (1957) original labeling of this factor as a "Superego Strength" source trait would seem to complete this consensus—except for the subtle interpretation he placed upon it: "Within the obvious varieties in super ego in our own culture, perhaps it is not fanciful to say that the common pattern which we find here in the young American male is a form of what Samuel Butler called the 'phillistine' pattern. It is direct and unsophisticated, with *values of simple achievement*—the well-known "success" of middle class and lower class ideology" (p.124, italics added).

The most persistent and persuasive advocate of an agentic interpretation of Factor III has been John Digman, whose investigations of teacher ratings of child personality provided a database ideally suited to the joint consideration of trait factor structure and academic achievement (Digman, 1963; Digman & Takemoto-Chock, 1981; Digman & Inouye, 1986). Digman's findings of substantial correlations of Factor III with academic performance and the similar results obtained by others (e.g., Wiggins, 1973, p. 357), led him to an explicitly agentic conception of Factor III as "Will to Achieve" (Digman, 1989; Digman & Takemoto-Chock, 1981).

McCrae's distinction between "proactive" and "inhibitive" manifestations of Conscientiousness has proven most useful in clarifying the conceptual differences between the many content facets of Factor III, that have been identified in the psychometric–trait literature (McCrae & Costa, 1987; McCrae & John, 1992). Proactive manifestations of Factor III involve the activation, direction, and organization of behavior toward the attainment of goals, as exemplified by such traits as achievement–striving and persistence. Inhibitive manifestations of Factor III involve the restraint and control of impulse in the service of goals and are best exemplified by such traits as cautiousness and dutifulness.

McCrae and John (1992) suggested that the term "Conscientiousness" might be preferred to other labels proposed for Factor III, because it connotes both inhibitive (e.g., governed by conscience) and proactive (e.g., diligent) aspects of this dimension, although the lexicographic support for this preference is not strong. In any event, McCrae's distinction is consistent with our assumption that agency and communion represent fundamental, social evaluative axes within all dimensions of the FFM. Our tentative judgments of their manifestations in some of the different content facets of Factor III are presented in Table 4.5. These judgments were guided by a distinction between self-discipline exercised in the pursuit of resources, power, or social status (*agency*) and self-discipline exercised in the pursuit of harmonious social relations (*communion*). Traits that would militate against the successful pursuit of these two enterprises are followed by a minus sign and traits that could arguably be classified under either or both enterprises are followed or preceded by an arrow. The instruments described in Table 4.5 (and Tables 4.6 and 4.7) were chosen because of their current prominence in the field and because each provides a suitably wide range of content facets for our purpose here.

Although we do not make any strong claims regarding the A and C assignments displayed in Table 4.5, and provide them mainly for illustrative purposes, we found it remarkably easy to agree on these assignments for this domain. Agentic and communal facets of Conscientiousness appear to be represented in approximately equal numbers in each of these influential FFM instruments, and the vast majority of them have a relatively clear connection to only one social metagoal, either agency or communion. Only two, closely related groups of facets proved difficult to classify: order (NEO-PI-R order, Revised Synonym Clusters [RSC] organization, and Multidimensional Personality Questionnaire [MPQ] makes detailed plans) and predictability (RSC predictability and Hogan Personality Inventory [HPI] not spontaneous). Being orderly, organized, and planful seemed to us just as likely to foster a social impression of responsibility (communion) as one of competence (agency).

TABLE 4.5. Classification of Conscientiousness Facets in Terms of Agency and Communion

Author(s)	Instrument	Scale	Agency	Communion
Costa & McCrae (1992)	NEO-PI-R	Conscientiousness	Achievement-striving Competence Discipline	Dutifulness Deliberation Order
Goldberg (1990)	RSC	Conscientiousness	Decisiveness Efficiency Persistence Precision Logic Nonconformity Dignity Frivolity (−) Aimlessness (−) Sloth (−)	Dependability Punctuality Thrift Caution Conventionality Forgetfulness (−) Organization Predictability
Hogan & Hogan (1992)	HPI	Prudence	Mastery Autonomy	Moralistic Virtuous Avoids trouble Impulse control Not spontaneous
Tellegen (1994)	MPQ	Control		Cautious Level-headed Reflective Makes detailed plans
		Traditionalism		Moralistic Endorses religion Positive regard for parents Endorses strict rearing Values "proper" conduct Opposes rebelliousness Condemns selfishness
		Achievement	Works hard Enjoys effort Welcomes difficulties Persistent Ambitious Perfectionistic	

Agency, Communion, and Neuroticism

From a lexical perspective, the factor of neuroticism has been characterized as "small" in relation to Extraversion, Agreeableness, and Conscientiousness, when the universe of content is restricted to ordinary-language dictionaries (Peabody & Goldberg, 1989). However, in the questionnaire realm in which psychological and psychiatric concepts have traditionally been given greater emphasis, the Neuroticism factor must be counted among the "Big Two" (Wiggins, 1968). The clusters of negative affects and cognitions that constitute Neuroticism tend to be more highly correlated than those within the other factors of the FFM, and for this reason high internal consistency and stability appear to be achieved (Costa & McCrae, 1992) at the occasional expense of discriminant validity (Wiggins, 1968). Within the area of psychopathology, the latter problem has been most acute in efforts to distinguish the facets of anxiety and depression (e.g., Dobson, 1985). Efforts to disentangle these two mood states and traits have emphasized their differential attributions or beliefs (Lazarus, 1966), their differential relations with positive affect (Tellegen, 1985), and their differential secondary loadings on other Big Five factors (Hofstee et al., 1992).

More critical to the problem of understanding Neuroticism as a dimension of the FFM is the problem of identifying the social contexts in which the various negative affects are embedded. The social evaluative implications of depression, anxiety, and anger may be discerned only within social contexts that are sufficiently specified to make clear about what or whom one is depressed, anxious, or angry.

Anxiety

The Minnesota Multiphasic Personality Inventory (MMPI) item, "I feel anxiety about something or someone almost all the time," appears in Taylor's (1953) Manifest Anxiety scale and is in some ways typical of the manner in which this construct is assessed via traditional questionnaires. The item refers to a global category of negative mood (anxiety) defined in the broadest conceivable dispositional language ("almost all the time"), with the vaguest conceivable contextual referents ("something or someone"). The social evaluative implications of anxiety may be discerned only within social contexts that are sufficiently specified to make clear what or whom one is anxious *about*.

Earlier in this chapter, a conceptual distinction was made between agentic and communal contexts for anxiety within Baumeister's (1990) exclusion theory. Situations involving possible loss of status give rise to agentic anxiety, and situations involving possible loss of love give rise to communal anxiety. Within the questionnaire realm, the Test Anxiety Scale (Mandler & Sarason, 1952) and the Audience Anxiety Scale (Paul, 1966) provide measures of agentic anxiety. Measures of communal anxiety are provided by the anxious attachment scale from Griffin and Bartholomew's (1994) Relationship Style Questionnaire and the mania (possessive, dependent love) scale from Hendrick and Hendrick's (1986) Love Attitudes Scale. Although numerous agentic and communal anxiety *items* may be found within existing questionnaires, such as the Fear of Negative Evaluation Scale (Watson & Friend, 1969); and the Self-Consciousness Scale (Fenigstein, Scheier, & Buss, 1975), a multiscale questionnaire designed specifically with reference to the agentic and communal distinction has yet to be constructed.

Depression

The MMPI item, "Most of the time I feel blue," expresses negative mood (depression) in broad dispositional language ("most of the time") in the absence of any indication of the circumstances or experiences that might be associated with the dysphoric affect. Recent research on depression has served to clarify the nature of some of these experiences and circumstances.

Blatt and Zuroff (1992) have provided a wide-ranging and highly integrative review of an extensive body of research that supports a distinction between two subtypes of depression based on different kinds of experiences that lead individuals to become depressed. The *autonomous* (self-critical) form of depression occurs in response to a perceived failure to maintain independence from others and to meet excessively high standards and ambitious goals. The *dependent* (sociotropic) form of depression occurs in response to a perceived threat of social rejection by others and fear of losing their help, care, support, and protection. This distinction has been made by investigators from a variety of theoretical perspectives (e.g., Arieti & Bemporad, 1978; Beck, 1983; Blatt, 1974; Bowlby, 1977), who use somewhat different terms but "all stress the importance of differentiating a depression focused on interpersonal issues such as dependency, helplessness, and feelings of loss and abandonment from a depression focused on issues of self-definition such as autonomy, self-criticism, and feelings of failure and guilt" (Blatt & Zuroff, 1992, p. 528).

Blatt and Zuroff (p. 530) discuss the similarity of the autonomy-dependency distinction to Bakan's (1966) distinction between *agency* and *communion*. In so doing, they relate the concept of "autonomy" to the personality dimensions of achievement (McClelland, 1986), power (Winter, 1973), and the interplay between the orthogonal dimensions of power and intimacy (McAdams, 1985b). From a structural perspective, this concept would appear to be complex, because psychometric measures of autonomy are generally uncorrelated with measures of power and control (agency), and are strongly negatively correlated with measures of nurturance (communion). However, the characterization of autonomous individuals as striving "for excessive achievement and perfection" (Blatt & Zuroff, 1992, p. 528) would seem to involve agentic facets of Conscientiousness (III), particularly achievement and competence (see Costa & McCrae, 1992, p. 73). The Depressive Experiences Questionnaire (DEQ; Blatt, D'Afflitti, & Quinlan, 1979) contains items of the latter type (e.g., "I find that I don't live up to my standards or ideals") on its autonomy (self-critical) scale, along with expressions of weakness, guilt, and lack of satisfaction in accomplishments. The concept of dependency is more clearly related to the metaconcept of communion. The DEQ dependency item, "Without support from others who are close to me I would be helpless," is representative of a scale that involves concerns about being alone, losing close friends, offending others, and being criticized by someone close. In Bowlby's (1977) terms, such individuals are "anxiously attached."

The two subtypes of depression that have figured prominently in recent research have not, as yet, been definitively related to the FFM. It would appear, however, that on a global level, a distinction is being made between threats to *self-esteem* and threats to *security* that involve at least four of the five factors of the model. The first two factors permit a distinction between autonomous and dependent individuals who are differentially vulnerable to the two types of depression. The third factor indexes the strivings for achievement and perfection of the autonomous type. The fourth factor could, in principle, permit a distinction between feelings of *worthlessness* associated with failed autonomy and feelings of *helplessness* associated with failed dependency. For the most part, FFM instruments have tended to strongly emphasize the former on this Neuroticism/Emotional Stability/Adjustment factor (e.g., Costa & McCrae, 1992; Goldberg, 1990). In contrast, the Adjustment factor of the HPI devotes three of its eight subscales to the communal characteristics of *good attachment, trust,* and *empathy* (Hogan & Hogan, 1992).

Anger

The MMPI item, "I sometimes feel like smashing things," is typical of the type of decontextualized frustration–anger item that most of us would admit to (scored *false* on the *K*-scale). The social–evaluative implications of such an item would vary considerably, however, as a function of what kinds of events or experiences provoke us to anger. Although there are excellent inventories of anger expression (e.g., A. H. Buss & Perry, 1992), there are few that attempt to specify the situations that provoke feelings of anger.

A recent study by Snell, McDonald, and Koch (1991) has taken a useful first step toward the specification of anger-provoking experiences. College students were asked to "write an essay describing what makes you feel angry," and their responses were classified into 48 categories by two coders. Brief descriptions and sample items from each of the 48 categories were provided to 19 psychologists, who grouped them into categories that were subjected to a multidimensional scaling analysis. A three-dimensional solution revealed what we would consider to be a clear dimension of *agentic frustration* and two somewhat related dimensions of *communal frustration*:

Dimension I. Anger-provoking experiences, "which thwart and constrain the actualization of an individual's personal ambitions, aims, goals, and values (e.g., academic problems, personal failure, foiled goals, inadequate planning"; pp. 1099–1100). Example: "I often get angry about my performance at school."

Dimension II. Anger-provoking experiences, "that are associated with public, social aspects of the self (e.g., rudeness, arrogance, hypocrisy"; p.1100). Example: "I get very angry about arrogant people."

Dimension III. "Events and experiences that are obviously lacking in interpersonal sensitivity (e.g., exploitation, criticism, jealousy"; p. 1100). Example: "I become very angry if I feel that someone is trying to take advantage of me."

The first dimension involves frustration over thwarted ambitions and strivings, which decreases feelings of *self-esteem*. The second and third dimensions involve situations of interpersonal effrontery and exploitation that are likely to destroy trust and thereby decrease feelings of *security*.

Although the distinction between agentic and communal components of Neuroticism has not been made by the major proponents of the FFM, the beginnings of such a conceptual distinction may be found within Tellegen's (1994) Multidimensional Personality Questionnaire (MPQ). The MPQ higher order factor of positive emotionality bifurcates into two factors of "agentic positive emotionality" (PEM-A) and "communal positive emotionality" (PEM-C; Tellegen & Waller, in press). Although both of these factors are loaded by well-being, PEM-A is defined by a loading of social closeness. The correlations of PEM-A and PEM-C with the negative emotionality facets of the MPQ were not available for the classifications made in Table 4.6.

For the reasons just elaborated, we did not expect many of the existing Neuroticism-facet scales to be easily classified as predominantly agentic or communal in their social evaluative implications. We decided to locate the "core" mood facets of anxiety and depression under agency because global, socially uncontextualized anxiety and depression markers of this sort tend to be substantially negatively correlated with interpersonal agency (e.g., dominance) and uncorrelated with interpersonal communion (e.g., nurturance). Global, socially undecontextualized markers of neurotic anger typically show the reverse pattern: negative correlations with communal interpersonal traits and very low or no correlation with agentic interpersonal traits. Anger-related facets have therefore been classified under communion. In factor studies of the MPQ scales, the alienation, aggression, and stress-reaction scales usually define a common factor of Negative Emotionality (Tellegen, 1994), the MPQ factor corresponding most closely to Neuroticism. The MPQ aggression scale has been included in Table 4.6 to reflect this fact. We suspect, however, that MPQ aggression is more highly related to Factor II (i.e., *Dis*agreeableness) than Factor IV, and that its high loading on Negative Emotionality may be due, in part, to underrepresentation of Factor II in the MPQ. For present purposes, we classify MPQ aggression with MPQ alienation as neurotic characteristics likely to impede communal social goals.

Agency, Communion, and Factor V

The most substantively contentious dimension of the FFM continues to be the fifth factor, as reflected in recent debates on this issue at conference symposia (e.g., Kihlstrom, 1992) and in a number of

TABLE 4.6. Classification of Neuroticism Facets in Terms of Agency and Communion

Author(s)	Instrument	Scale	Agency	Communion
Costa & McCrae (1992)	NEO-PI-R	Neuroticism	Depression (−) Vulnerability (−) Self-consciousness (−) Anxiety (−) Impulsivity (−)	Hostility (−)
Goldberg (1990)	RSC	Emotional Stability	Independence Insecurity (−) Gullibility (−) Fear (−)	Envy (−) Intrusiveness (−) Instability (−) Placidity
Hogan & Hogan (1992)	HPI	Adjustment	Not anxious No guilt No somatic complaints	Empathy Trusting Even tempered Good attachment Calmness
Tellegen (1994)	MPQ	Stress Reaction	Tense, nervous (−) Vulnerable, sensitive (−) Worry-prone, anxious (−) Easily upset (−) Prone to feel guilty (−) Unexplainable negative emotions (−)	
		Alienation		Pushed around (−) Target of malevolence (−) Betrayed, deceived (−) Exploited (−) Victim of false rumors (−) Unlucky (−)
		Aggression		Enjoys distressing others (−) Victimizes for own gain (−) Vengeful, vindictive (−) Enjoys witnessing violence (−) Physically aggressive (−)

academic journals (e.g., De Raad & van Heck, 1994). These debates center on whether the lexical fifth factor reflects social judgments of intellectual ability, competency, or sophistication that would suggest an "intelligence," "intellect," or "imagination" interpretation (e.g., Goldberg, 1981; Peabody & Goldberg, 1989; Saucier, 1992), or whether interpretations of Factor V should incorporate a broad range of questionnaire data, and cognitive–structural and motivational assumptions that together suggest an alternative view of Factor V as "Openness to Experience" (McCrae, 1990; 1994; McCrae & Costa, 1985, in press).

Both Intellect and Openness conceptions of Factor V share a focus on cognitive dispositions, particularly those related to divergent thinking such as curiosity, creativity, and imaginativeness. However, as Trapnell (1994) recently noted, Intellect conceptions of Factor V emphasize *competence*, whereas Openness conceptions stress motives, interests, and egalitarian values associated with *liberalism*. On this view, the social implications of prototypic Intellect terms (e.g., *intelligent, smart, brainy, knowledgeable, clever*) are mainly *agentic* in that they connote competency, mastery, superiority, or leadership, qualities predictive of social ascendancy or status. The social implications of prototypic Openness terms (e.g., *aesthetically sensitive, reflective, imaginative, empathic, open-minded*) are mainly *communal*, in that they connote qualities associated with interpersonal warmth, acceptance, and tolerance. In the context in which we have been using the terms, Openness may be viewed as a "feminine" and Intellect as a "masculine" conception of Factor V, and the Openness versus Intellect debate thus becomes one over the "heart" and "mind" of Factor V (Trapnell, 1994).

Agentic Factor V

Three lines of evidence provide support for an agentic conception of Factor V: (1) consistent, positive correlations between Factor V and psychometric indicators of intellectual performance (McCrae, 1987; McCrae & Costa, 1985; Hogan & Hogan, 1992), and positive correlations between Factor V and other objective indicators of intellectual performance, achievement, and status (Hogan, 1986; Hogan & Hogan, 1992); (2) consistent, positive correlations between Intellect or Openness factors and Factor I, Surgency/Extraversion, whether measured by adjectives (Goldberg, 1990; Trapnell & Wiggins, 1990) or questionnaires (Costa & McCrae, 1992; Hogan & Hogan, 1992); and (3) the wide range of agency-related trait measures positively correlated with Factor V, including Holland's (1973, 1985b) enterprising vocational type; the assured–dominant scale of Wiggins's (1995) IAS (Hogan & Hogan, 1992); the ambition and managerial potential scales of the Hogan Personality Inventory (Hogan & Hogan, 1992), and the dominance, capacity for status, achievement via conformance, and achievement via independence scales of Gough's (1987) California Psychological Inventory (e.g., Botwin & Buss, 1989; Hogan & Hogan, 1992; McCrae, Costa, & Piedmont, 1993).

A close association between agentic interpersonal traits and intellect was assumed by Cattell (1945) in an early version of his 35 bipolar rating scales, the scales that were so influential in the development of the FFM. As noted by John, Angleitner, and Ostendorf (1988), Cattell's item 35 originally contrasted "sophisticated, intelligent, and assertive" with "simple, stupid, and submissive." Apparently, Cattell considered assertiveness and intellectual sophistication to be empirically so closely associated that markers for them could be collapsed into a single scale. Although references to sophistication and intelligence were later eliminated from this item (Cattell, 1947), and the later version was adopted by subsequent users of the scales (e.g., Fiske, 1949; Tupes & Christal, 1961/1992; Norman, 1963), the factor structure of Cattell's 16 PF Questionnaire does appear to support Cattell's early conjoining of assertiveness with aspects of Factor V. The higher order factor of the 16 PF that corresponds most closely to Factor V of the FFM is the "independence" factor, defined by primary factors M (imaginative vs. practical), Q (experimenting vs. conservative), and E (dominance vs. submissiveness) (Cattell, Eber, & Tatsuoka, 1970).

Communal Factor V

Closely related to this openness to inner and outer experience in general is an openness to and an acceptance of other individuals. As a client moves toward being able to accept his own experience, he also moves toward the acceptance of the experiences of others.
—ROGERS (1961, pp. 174–175)

The communal implications of openness are evident across a wide range of psychological research literatures. In vocational psychology, a close association between artistic and social-welfare occupational interests is well known and perhaps best exemplified by the adjacent locations of social and artistic vocational types in Holland's (1973, 1985b) circumplex model of vocational interests. In sociology and political psychology, a close association between communion and Factor V is evident in the well-known association between liberalism and occupation. Whereas police, engineers, tradespersons, farmers, and accountants are among the most sociopolitical conservative vocational groups in Western society, artists, scientists, educators, and journalists are typically the most liberal (e.g., Campbell & Rossman, 1972). The aesthetic and theoretical value orientations—the hallmark of high Factor V individuals— of the latter, prototypically liberal groups clearly distinguish them from the pragmatic and economic value orientations of the former, more conservative ones. One might interpret both the egalitarian social ethos of liberals (i.e., ethnic, religious, and sexual tolerance) and their artistic and intellectual vocational choices as arising from a common source: values, interests, and attitudes arising from stable personality differences in cognitive and emotional openness.

Agentic and communal classifications of Factor V scales from four instruments are presented in Table 4.7. As before, no strong claims are made for these judgments, and they are presented for purposes of illustration only. It would appear from Table 4.7 that the HPI and RSC Factor V scales focus almost exclusively on agentic features, and that the NEO-PI-R scales focus more on communal features.

Item clusters from the absorption and harmavoidance scales also appear in Table 4.7. Previous structural analyses of the MPQ failed to reveal a higher order factor corresponding to Factor V; instead, absorption and harmavoidance loaded on dimensions corresponding to other FFM dimensions (e.g., Tellegen & Waller, in press, Table 3). However, other lines of evidence suggested that MPQ absorption and harmavoidance are best designated as Factor V scales within the FFM framework (e.g., Costa & McCrae, 1988; McCrae & Costa, 1985; Tellegen & Waller, in press, Table 6; Trapnell, 1992).

Within the present schema, we considered the facets of harmavoidance to be inhibitive of agentic traits such as curiosity and openness to actions. Absorption was classified as communal for reasons well expressed by Tellegen and Atkinson (1974): "The motivational–affective component [of absorption] would seem to consist in a sentient and tolerant 'openness to experience' (Fitzgerald, 1966),

TABLE 4.7. Classification of Factor V Facets in Terms of Agency and Communion

Author(s)	Instrument	Scale	Agency	Communion
Costa & McCrae (1992)	NEO-PI-R	Openness	Ideas Actions	Aesthetics Feelings Values Fantasy
Goldberg (1990)	RSC	Intellect	Intelligence Intellectuality Depth Sophistication Shallowness (−) Imperceptiveness (−) Stupidity (−) Curiosity	Creativity Unimagina- tiveness (−)
Hogan & Hogan (1992)	HPI	Intellectance	Generates ideas Science Curiosity Thrill-seeking Intellectual games	Culture
		School Success	Math ability Good memory Education	Reading

Tellegen (1994)	MPQ	Absorption		Evocative stimuli
				Involving stimuli
				Expanded
				  awareness
				Thinks in images
				Cross-modal
				  experiences
				Can relive past
				Vivid imagination
				Altered awareness
				Absorbed in
				  thoughts

		Harm-avoidance(−)	Dislikes risky
			  adventures (−)
			Avoids disaster
			  areas (−)
			Dislikes
			  emergencies (−)
			Avoids injury (−)	

a desire and readiness for object relationships temporary or lasting that permit experiences of deep involvement. The content of several Absorption markers, including the Openness to Experience and Devotion–Trust scales, is suggestive in this respect" (p. 275).

Higher Order Factors in the Five-Factor Model

Digman's (1991) comprehensive investigation of higher order factors of the FFM yielded results that are highly consistent with the dyadic–interactional perspective. Two higher order factors were clearly evident in 11 diverse studies of children, adolescents, and adults. The first factor (Alpha) was loaded by the primary factors of Agreeableness, Conscientiousness, and Neuroticism (the latter loading negatively). Digman interpreted this factor within the context of theories of socialization that stress the reduction of hostility and aggression, the development of conscience, and the development of impulse restraint, all in preparation for group living. The second factor (Beta) was loaded by Extraversion and Intellect/Openness, and was interpreted as personal growth versus personal constriction in line with the writings of Rogers (1961) and Maslow (1971). In this context, Digman suggested that the primary factors (I and V) underlying this higher order factor might be better construed as Surgency and Openness to Experience, respectively.

In his more general consideration of personality theorists who have employed both of these higher order constructs as fundamental distinctions (see Table 4.3 in the present chapter), Digman acknowledged the heuristic value of an agency (Factor Beta) and communion (Factor Alpha) formulation and provided a felicitous characterization of these metaconcepts: "These two factors, at the highest level of abstraction in the lexicon of personality constructs, appear to reflect some basic themes of human nature—a natural tendency to organize in hierarchical fashion and a value system that promoted reciprocal friendly alliances, the assumption of responsibility, and the display of fortitude under stress" (p. 15).

Digman's characterizations of the social forces operative in a society appear to be very close to our own. Although his conclusions are based on factor analysis and are thereby possibly open to criticism on methodological grounds, such issues should not detract from the advantages of a guiding theoretical orientation that postulates what the structure of personality might be, independent of any particular method of data analysis. That the components of both the FFM and the Big Five are interrelated seems evident (Block, 1995; Hofstee et al., 1992). On the level of ordinary language usage, the two "circumplex factors," despite their potency, cannot be "walled off" from the remaining three (De Raad, in press). Some rationale for this fact of nature is clearly needed.

We have found the FFM to be an especially useful framework for "grounding"our metapsychological speculations about the role of agency and communion in society. Equally important, however, has been the opportunity this model has provided us for "communication" with some of the leading figures in personality psychology, whose diverse and highly specialized programs of research might otherwise have proven less permeable to interchanges of ideas.

Notes

1. Spence and Helmreich (1978, pp. 14–15) make the important point that early role theorists, such as Parsons and Bales, distinguish between sex-role behavior (e.g., leading others) and dispositional properties of the behaving organism (e.g., the trait of dominance). This distinction between role taking and role playing (Horrocks & Jackson, 1972) helps avoid the confusion generated by the all-purpose label of "sex role" that has characterized the recent literature on this topic (see also Spence, 1985).

2. McAdams (1985b) reported difficulties in interpreting the protocols of subjects whose life stories were based on characters who lacked both agency and communion (pp. 202–203) and suspected that such imagoes might be equally difficult to apply to the study of interpersonal relationships (1985a, p. 136). Similar interpretive ambiguities were encountered by Bem (1977) with "undifferentiated" subjects who were low on both masculinity and femininity. These difficulties may reflect the shortcomings of a *unipolar* structural model for representing agency and communion (Wiggins, 1991a, Fig. 2 and pp. 105–106) rather than the absence of "passivity" and "dissociation" in life stories.

3. Denying love to self and denying love to another are similarly related.

4. In what is from our perspective a related contribution, Andrews (1989) discusses differences among schools of psychotherapy within the framework of Leary's (1957) interpersonal circumplex model.

5. Anxiety is dealt with by the "self-system" (not to be confused with the personification of self). Ford and Urban (1963) provide one of the clearest discussions of this highly abstract concept that "referred to all the behaviors the child acquires in the course of his interpersonal relationships which perform the function of avoiding or minimizing the occurrence of anxiety.

In other terms, the concept referred to the group of avoidance behaviors acquired in relation to people" (p. 543).

6. Sullivan's account of the origins of anxiety appears to be a source of embarrassment for even his most enthusiastic supporters (e.g., Chapman, 1976; Chrzanowski, 1977; Mullahy, 1970). Levenson (1991) observed that Sullivan's formulation of anxiety represented a retreat from an operationalized system based on an interpersonal communication model of information processing to the earlier conception of "a mysterious energic ether" of psychoanalytic metapsychology (p. 147). Levenson also provided a sympathetic and penetrating analysis of aspects of Sullivan's personality that may have contributed to this conceptual "slippage."

7. We are most grateful to Victor R. Lovell for calling this material to our attention (personal communication, August 1991).

8. Wiggins's ideas about space travel were more strongly influenced by early Buck Rogers films than by *Star Trek.*

References

Adler, A. (1964). On the origin of the striving for superiority and of social interest. In H. L. Ansbacher & R. R. Ansbacher (Eds.), *Alfred Adler: Superiority and social interest* (pp. 29–40). New York: Viking Press. (Original work published 1933)

Alden, L. E., Wiggins, J. S., & Pincus, A. L. (1990). Construction of circumplex scales for the Inventory of Interpersonal Problems. *Journal of Personality Assessment, 55,* 521–536.

American Psychiatric Association. (1980). *Diagnostic and statistical manual of mental disorders* (3rd ed.). Washington, DC: Author.

Andrews, J. D. W. (1989). Integrating visions of reality: Interpersonal diagnosis and the existential vision. *American Psychologist, 44,* 803–817.

Angyal, A. (1941). *Foundations for a science of personality.* New York: Viking Press.

Arieti, S., & Bemporad, J. (1978). *Severe and mild depression: The psychotherapeutic approach.* New York: Basic Books.

Bakan, D. (1966). *The duality of human existence: Isolation and communion in Western man.* Boston: Beacon.

Bales, R. F. (1950). *Interaction process analysis: A method for the study of small groups.* Cambridge, MA: Addison-Wesley.

Baumeister, R. F. (1990). Anxiety and deconstruction: On escaping the self. In J. M. Olson & M. P. Zanna (Eds.), *Self-inference processes: The Ontario Symposium* (Vol. 6, pp. 259–291). Hillsdale, NJ: Erlbaum.

Beck, A. T. (1983). Cognitive therapy of depression: New perspectives. In P. J. Clayton & J.E. Barrett (Eds.), *Treatment of depression: old controversies and new approaches* (pp. 265–290). New York: Raven Press.

Bem, S. L. (1977). On the utility of alternative scoring procedures for assessing psychological androgyny. *Journal of Consulting and Clinical Psychology, 45,* 196–205.

Benjamin, L. S. (1993). *Interpersonal diagnosis and treatment of personality disorders.* New York: Guilford Press.

Berne, E. (1972). *What do you say after you say hello?* New York: Grove Press.

Blatt, S. J. (1974). Levels of object representation in anaclitic and introjective depression. *The Psychoanalytic Study of the Child, 24,* 107–157.

Blatt, S. J., D'Afflitti, J. P., & Quinlan, D. M. (1979). *Depressive Experiences Questionnaire.* Unpublished manuscript, Yale University, New Haven, CT.

Blatt, S. J., & Zuroff, D. C. (1992). Interpersonal relatedness and self-definition: Two prototypes for depression. *Clinical Psychology Review, 12,* 527–562.

Block, J. (1995). A contrarian view of the five-factor approach to personality disorder. *Psychological Bulletin, 117,* 187–215.

Botwin, M. D., & Buss, D. M. (1989). Structure of act–report data: Is the five-factor model of personality recaptured? *Journal of Personality and Social Psychology, 56,* 988–1001.

Bowlby, J. (1969). *Attachment and loss: Vol. I. Attachment.* New York: Basic Books.

Bowlby, J. (1973). *Attachment and loss: Vol. II. Separation anxiety and anger.* New York: Basic Books.

Bowlby, J. (1977). The making and breaking of affectional bonds: 1. Etiology and psychopathology in light of attachment theory. *British Journal of Psychiatry, 130,* 201–210.

Browne, M. W. (1992). Circumplex models for correlation matrices. *Psychometrika, 57,* 469–497.

Buss, A. H., & Perry, M. (1992). The Aggression Questionnaire. *Journal of Personality and Social Psychology, 63,* 452–459.

Buss, D. M. (1986). Can social science be anchored in evolutionary biology? *Review of European Social Science, 24,* 41–53.

Buss, D. M. (1989). Sex differences in human mate preferences: Evolutionary hypotheses tested in 37 cultures. *Behavioral and Brain Sciences, 12,* 1–49.

Buss, D. M. (1991a). Conflict in married couples: Personality predictors of anger and upset. *Journal of Personality, 59,* 663–688.

Buss, D. M. (1991b). Evolutionary personality psychology. In M. R. Rosenzweig & L. W. Porter (Eds.), *Annual review of psychology* (Vol. 41, pp. 459–491). Palo Alto CA: Annual Reviews.

Buss, D. M. (1994). *The evolution of desire: Strategies of human mating.* New York: Basic Books.

Buss, D. M. (1995). Evolutionary psychology: A new paradigm for psychological science. *Psychological Inquiry, 6,* 1–30.

Buss, D. M., & Craik, K. H. (1983). Act prediction and the conceptual analysis of personality scales: Indices of act density, bipolarity, and extensity. *Journal of Personality and Social Psychology, 45,* 1081–1095.

Buss, D. M., & Schmitt, D. P. (1993). Sexual strategies theory: An evolutionary perspective on human mating. *Psychological Review, 100,* 204–232.

Campbell, D. P., & Rossman, J. E. (1972, September). *A liberalism–conservatism scale for the Strong Vocational Interest Blank.* Paper presented at the annual meeting of the American Psychological Association, Honolulu, HI.

Cannon, W. B. (1939). *The wisdom of the body* (rev. ed.). New York: Norton.

Cantor, N., & Mischel, W. (1979). Prototypes in person perception. In L. Berkowitz (Ed.), *Advances in experimental social psychology* (Vol. 12, pp. 3–53). New York: Academic Press.

Carson, R. C. (1969). *Interaction concepts of personality.* Chicago: Aldine.

Carson, R. C. (1979). Personality and exchange in developing relationships. In R. L. Burgess & T. L. Huston (Eds.), *Social exchange in developing relationships* (pp. 247–269). New York: Academic Press.

Carson, R. C. (1989). Personality. In M. R. Rosenzweig & L. W. Porter (Eds.), *Annual review of psychology* (Vol. 40, pp. 227–248). Palo Alto, CA: Annual Reviews.

Carson, R. C. (1991). The social–interactional viewpoint. In M. Hersen, A. Kazdin, & A. Bellack (Eds.), *The clinical psychology handbook* (2nd ed., pp. 185–199). Elmsford, NY: Pergamon Press.

Cattell, R. B. (1945). The description of personality: Principles and findings in a factor analysis. *American Journal of Psychology, 58*, 69–90.

Cattell, R. B. (1947). Confirmation and clarification of primary personality factors. *Psychometrika, 12*, 197–220.

Cattell, R. B. (1957). *Personality and motivation structure and measurement.* New York: World Book.

Cattell, R. B., Eber, H. W., & Tatsuoka, M. M. (1970). *Handbook for the Sixteen Personality Factor Questionnaire (16 PF).* Champaign, IL: Institute for Personality and Ability Testing.

Chapman, A. H. (1976). *Harry Stack Sullivan: His life and work.* New York: Putnam.

Chrzanowski, G. (1977). *Interpersonal approaches to psychoanalysis: A contemporary view of Harry Stack Sullivan.* New York: Gardner Press.

Cohen, M. B. (1953). Introduction. In H. S. Sullivan, *The interpersonal theory of psychiatry* (pp. xi–xviii). New York: Norton.

Costa, P. T., Jr., & McCrae, R. R. (1988). From catalogue to classification: Murray's needs and the five-factor model. *Journal of Personality and Social Psychology, 55*, 258–265.

Costa, P. T., Jr., & McCrae, R. R. (1992). *NEO PI-R: Professional manual.* Odessa, FL: Psychological Assessment Resources.

Costa, P. T., Jr., & Widiger, T. A. (Eds.). (1994). *Personality disorders and the five-factor model of personality.* Washington, DC: American Psychological Association.

Craik, K. H. (1986). Personality research methods: An historical perspective. *Journal of Personality, 54*, 18–51.

Darwin, C. (1859). *On the origin of the species by means of natural selection, or Preservation of favored races in the struggle for life.* London: Murray.

Darwin, C. (1871). *The descent of man and selection in relation to sex.* London: Murray.

De Raad, B. (in press.). The psycho-lexical approach to the structure of interpersonal traits. *European Journal of Personality.*

De Raad, B., & van Heck, G. L. (Eds.). (1994). Special issue: The fifth of the Big Five. *European Journal of Personality, 8.*

Digman, J. M. (1963). Principal dimensions of child personality as inferred from teachers' judgments. *Child Development, 34,* 43–60.

Digman, J. M. (1989). Five robust trait dimensions: Development, stability, and utility. *Journal of Personality, 57,* 195–214.

Digman, J. M. (1991). The Big Five: Up, down, and beyond. In S. Strack (Chair), *Beyond the Big Five.* Symposium at the 99th annual meeting of the American Psychological Association, San Francisco, CA.

Digman, J. M., & Inouye, J. (1986). Further specification of the five robust factors of personality. *Journal of Personality and Social Psychology, 50,* 116–123.

Digman, J. M., & Takemoto-Chock, N. K. (1981). Factors in the natural language of personality: Re-analysis, comparison, and interpretation of six major studies. *Multivariate Behavioral Research, 16,* 149–170.

Dobson, K. S. (1985). The relationship between anxiety and depression. *Clinical Psychology Review, 5,* 307–324.

Eagly, A. H. (1987). *Sex differences in social behavior: A social-role interpretation.* Hillsdale, NJ: Erlbaum.

Eldridge, S. (1925). *The organization of life.* New York: Crowell.

Erikson, E. H. (1950). *Childhood and society.* New York: Norton.

Erikson, E. H. (1959). Identity and the life cycle: Selected papers. *Psychological Issues, 1*(1), 5–165.

Fairbairn, W. R. D. (1952). *Psychoanalytic studies of the personality.* London: Routledge & Kegan Paul.

Fenigstein, A., Scheier, M., & Buss, A. (1975). Public and private self-consciousness: Assessment and theory. *Journal of Consulting and Clinical Psychology, 43,* 522–527.

Fiske, D. W. (1949). Consistency of the factorial structures of personality ratings from different sources. *Journal of Abnormal and Social Psychology, 44,* 329–344.

Fitzgerald, E. T. (1966). Measurable components of openness to experience: A study of regression in the service of the ego. *Journal of Personality and Social Psychology, 4,* 655–663.

Foa, E. B., & Foa, U. G. (1976). Resource theory of social exchange. In J. W. Thibaut, J. T. Spence, & R. C. Carson (Eds.), *Contemporary topics in social psychology.* Morristown, NJ: General Learning Press.

Foa, E. B., & Foa, U. G. (1980). Resource theory. In K. J. Gergen, M. S. Greenberg, & R. H. Willis (Eds.), *Social exchange: Advances in theory and research* (pp. 77–94). New York: Plenum Press.

Foa, U. G. (1965). New developments in facet design and analysis. *Psychological Review, 72,* 262–274.

Foa, U. G., Converse, J. M., Jr., Törnblom, K. Y., & Foa, E. B. (1993). *Resource theory: Explorations and applications.* Orlando, FL: Academic Press.

Foa, U. G., & Foa, E. B. (1974). *Societal structures of the mind.* Springfield, IL: Thomas.

Ford, D. H., & Urban, H. B. (1963). *Systems of psychotherapy: A comparative study.* New York: Wiley.

Freedman, M. B., Leary, T. F., Ossorio, A. G., & Coffey, H. S. (1951). The interpersonal dimension of personality. *Journal of Personality, 20,* 143–161.

Freud, S. (1964). New introductory lectures on psychoanalysis. In J. Strachey (Ed.), *The standard edition of the complete works of Sigmund Freud* (Vol. 22, pp. 3–182). London: Hogarth Press. (Original work published 1933)

Fromm, E. (1941). *Escape from freedom.* New York: Avon Books.

Gifford, R. (1991). Mapping nonverbal behavior on the Interpersonal Circle. *Journal of Personality and Social Psychology, 61,* 279–288.

Gilligan, C. (1982). *In a different voice: Psychological theory and women's development.* Cambridge: Harvard University Press.

Goldberg, L. R. (1981). Language and individual differences: The search for universals in personality lexicons. In L. W. Wheeler (Ed.), *Review of personality and social psychology* (Vol. 2, pp. 141–165). Beverly Hills, CA: Sage.

Goldberg, L. R. (1982). From Ace to Zombie: Some explorations in the language of personality. In C. D. Spielberger & J. N. Butcher (Eds.), *Advances in personality assessment* (Vol. 1, pp. 203–234). Hillsdale, NJ: Erlbaum.

Goldberg, L. R. (1990). An alternative description of personality: The Big Five factor structure. *Journal of Personality and Social Psychology, 59,* 1216–1229.

Gough, H. G. (1987). *California Psychological Inventory administrator's guide.* Palo Alto, CA: Consulting Psychologists Press.

Griffin, D. W., & Bartholomew, K. (1994). The metaphysics of measurement: The case of adult attachment. In K. Bartholomew & D. Perlman (Eds.), *Advances in personal relationships: Attachment processes in adulthood* (Vol. 5, pp. 17–52). London: Jessica Kingsley.

Gurtman, M. B. (1991). Evaluating the interpersonalness of personality scales. *Personality and Social Psychology Bulletin, 17,* 670–677.

Gurtman, M. B. (1992a). Construct validity of interpersonal personality measures: The Interpersonal Circumplex as a nomological net. *Journal of Personality and Social Psychology, 63,* 105–118.

Gurtman, M. B. (1992b). Trust, distrust, and interpersonal problems: A circumplex analysis. *Journal of Personality and Social Psychology, 62,* 989–1002.

Gurtman, M. B. (1994). The circumplex as a tool for studying normal and abnormal personality: A methodological primer. In S. Strack & M. Lorr (Eds.), *Differentiating normal and abnormal personality* (pp. 243–263). New York: Springer.

Gurtman, M. B., & Balakrishnan, J. D. (1994). *Circular measurement redux: The analysis and interpretation of circular interpersonal profiles.* Unpublished manuscript, University of Wisconsin at Parkside.

Guttman, L. (1954). A new approach to factor analysis: The radex. In P. R. Lazarsfeld (Ed.), *Mathematical thinking in the social sciences* (pp. 258–348). Glencoe, IL: Free Press.

Hartmann, H., & Lowenstein, R. M. (1964). Notes on the superego. *Psychological Issues, 4,* 144–181.

Hendrick, C., & Hendrick, S. (1986). A theory and method of love. *Journal of Personality and Social Psychology, 50,* 392–402.

Hofstee, W. K. B., De Raad, B., & Goldberg, L. R. (1992). Integration of the Big Five and circumplex approaches to trait structure. *Journal of Personality and Social Psychology, 63,* 146–163.

Hogan, R. (1983). A socioanalytic theory of personality. In M. M. Page (Ed.), *1982 Nebraska symposium on motivation: Personality–current theory and research* (pp. 58–89). Lincoln: University of Nebraska Press.

Hogan, R. (1986). *Hogan Personality Inventory manual.* Minneapolis, MN: National Computer Systems.

Hogan, R., & Hogan, J. (1992). *Hogan Personality Inventory manual.* Tulsa, OK: Hogan Assessment Systems.

Holland, J. L. (1973). *Making vocational choices: A theory of careers.* Engelwood Cliffs, NJ: Prentice-Hall.

Holland, J. L. (1985a). *Professional manual for the Vocational Preference Inventory.* Odessa, FL: Psychological Assessment Resources.

Holland, J. L. (1985b). *Making vocational choices: A theory of vocational personalities and work environments* (2nd ed.). Englewood Cliffs, NJ: Prentice-Hall.

Horney, K. (1937). *The neurotic personality of our time.* New York: Norton.

Horowitz, L. M. (1979). On the cognitive structure of interpersonal problems treated in psychotherapy. *Journal of Consulting and Clinical Psychology, 47,* 5–15.

Horowitz, L. M., Rosenberg, S. E., Baer, B. A., Ureno, G., & Villasenor, V. S. (1988). Inventory of Interpersonal Problems: Psychometric properties and clinical applications. *Journal of Consulting and Clinical Psychology, 56,* 885–892.

Horrocks, J. E., & Jackson, D. W. (1972). *Self and role: A theory of self-process and role behavior.* Boston: Houghton Mifflin.

Hui, C. H., & Triandis, H. C. (1986). Individualism–collectivism: A study of cross-cultural researchers. *Journal of Cross-Cultural Psychology, 17,* 225–248.

Ilchman, W. F., & Uphoff, N. T. (1969). *The political economy of change.* Berkeley: University of California Press.

John, O. P., Angleitner, A. & Ostendorf, F. (1988). The lexical approach to personality: A historical review of trait taxonomic research. *European Journal of Personality, 2,* 171–203.

Johnson, J. A., & Ostendorf, F. (1993). Clarification of the five-factor model with the abridged Big Five dimensional circumplex. *Journal of Personality and Social Psychology, 65,* 563–576.

Jung, C. G. (1943). The psychology of the unconscious. In *Collected works* (Vol. 7, pp. 3–117). Princeton, NJ: Princeton University Press.

Kenrick, D. T. (1989). A biosocial perspective on mates and traits: Reuniting personality and social psychology. In D. M. Buss & N. Cantor (Eds.), *Personality psychology: Recent trends and emerging directions* (pp. 308–319). New York: Springer.

Kenrick, D. T., & Keefe, R. C. (1989). Time to integrate sociobiology and social psychology. *Behavioral and Brain Sciences, 12,* 24–26.

Kiesler, D. J. (1979). An interpersonal communication analysis of relationships in psychotherapy. *Psychiatry, 42,* 299–311.

Kiesler, D. J. (1982). Interpersonal theory for personality and psychotherapy. In J. C. Anchin & D. J. Kiesler (Eds.), *Handbook of interpersonal psychotherapy* (pp. 3–24). New York: Pergamon Press.

Kiesler, D. J. (1983). The 1982 Interpersonal Circle: A taxonomy for complementarity in human transactions. *Psychological Review, 90,* 185–214.

Kiesler, D. J. (1986). The 1982 Interpersonal Circle: An analysis of DSM-III personality disorders. In T. Millon & G.L. Klerman (Eds.), *Contemporary directions in psychopathology: Toward the DSM-IV* (pp. 571–597). New York: Guilford Press.

Kiesler, D. J. (1987). *Manual for the Impact Message Inventory: Research edition.* Palo Alto, CA: Consulting Psychologists Press.

Kiesler, D. J. (1988). *Therapeutic metacommunication: Therapist impact disclosure as feedback in psychotherapy.* Palo Alto, CA: Consulting Psychologists Press.

Kiesler, D. J., & Schmidt, J. A. (1991). *The Impact Message Inventory: Form IIA Octant Scale Version.* Richmond: Virginia Commonwealth University.

Kihlstrom, J. F. (1992, August). *Intellectance and openness in the "Big Five" personality structure.* Symposium at the annual convention of the American Psychological Association, Washington, DC.

LaForge, R. (1963, April). *Interpersonal domains or interpersonal levels? A validation study of Leary's "MMPI Level I Indices."* Paper presented at the annual meeting of the Western Psychological Association, Santa Monica, CA.

LaForge, R. (1977). *Using the ICL: 1976.* Mill Valley, CA: Author.

LaForge, R., Leary, T. F., Naboisek, H., Coffey, H. S., & Freedman, M. B. (1954). The interpersonal dimension of personality: II. An objective study of repression. *Journal of Personality, 23,* 129–153.

Lazarus, R. (1966). *Psychological stress and the coping process.* New York: McGraw-Hill.

Leary, T. (1956). *Multilevel measurement of interpersonal behavior.* Berkeley, CA: Psychological Consultation Service.

Leary, T. (1957). *Interpersonal diagnosis of personality.* New York: Ronald Press.

Levenson, E. A. (1991). Harry Stack Sullivan: The web and the spider. In A.

H. Feiner (Ed.), *The purloined self: Interpersonal perspectives in psychoanalysis* (pp. 135–149). New York: W. A. White Institute.

Loevinger, J. (1957). Objective tests as instruments of psychological theory. *Psychological Reports, 3*(Monograph No. 9), 635–694.

Loranger, A. (1988). *Personality Disorder Examination (PDE) manual.* White Plains, NY: Cornell University Medical College, Department of Psychiatry.

Lorr, M., & McNair, D. M. (1967). *The Interpersonal Behavior Inventory: Form 4.* Washington, DC: Catholic University of America.

Lukes, S. (1973). *Individualism.* Oxford: Blackwell.

Mandler, G., & Sarason, S. B. (1952). A study of anxiety and learning. *Journal of Abnormal and Social Psychology, 47,* 166–173.

Markus, H., & Nurius, P. (1986). Possible selves. *American Psychologist, 41,* 954–969.

Maslow, A. H. (1971). *The farther reaches of human nature.* New York: Viking.

McAdams, D. P. (1985a). The "imago": A key narrative component of identity. In P. Shaver (Ed.), *Review of personality and social psychology* (Vol. 6, pp. 115–141). Beverly Hills, CA: Sage.

McAdams, D. P. (1985b). *Power, intimacy, and the life story: Personological inquiries into identity.* New York: Guilford Press.

McAdams, D. P. (1989). *Intimacy: The need to be close.* New York: Doubleday.

McAdams, D. P. (1990). *The person: An introduction to personality psychology.* New York: Harcourt Brace Jovanovich.

McAdams, D. P. (1991). Self and story. In A. J. Stewart, J. M. Healy, Jr., & D. Ozer (Eds.), *Perspectives in personality* (Vol. 3, pp. 133–159). London: Jessica Kingsley.

McAdams, D. P. (1993). *The stories we live by: Personal myths and the making of self.* New York: William Morrow.

McClelland, D. C. (1986). Some reflections on the two psychologies of love. *Journal of Personality, 54,* 334–353.

McCrae, R. R. (1987). Creativity, divergent thinking, and openness to experience. *Journal of Personality and Social Psychology, 52,* 1258–1265.

McCrae, R. R. (1990). Traits and trait names: How well is Openness represented in natural language? *European Journal of Personality, 4,* 119–129.

McCrae, R. R. (1994). Openness to experience: Expanding the boundaries of Factor V. *European Journal of Personality, 8,* 251–272.

McCrae, R. R., & Costa, P. T., Jr. (1985). Openness to experience. In R. Hogan, & W. H. Jones (Eds.), *Perspectives in personality* (Vol. 1, pp. 145–172). Greenwich, CT: JAI Press.

McCrae, R. R., & Costa, P. T., Jr. (1987). Validation of the five-factor model across instruments and observers. *Journal of Personality and Social Psychology, 52,* 81–90.

McCrae, R. R., & Costa, P. T., Jr. (1989). The structure of interpersonal traits: Wiggins' circumplex and the five-factor model. *Journal of Personality and Social Psychology, 56,* 586–595.

McCrae, R. R., & Costa, P.T., Jr. (in press). Conceptions and correlates of openness to experience. In R. Hogan, J. A. Johnson, & S. R. Briggs (Eds.), *Handbook of personality psychology*. Orlando, FL: Academic Press.

McCrae, R. R., Costa, P. T., Jr., & Piedmont, R. L. (1993). Folk concepts, natural language, and psychological constructs: The California Psychological Inventory and the five-factor model. *Journal of Personality, 61*, 1–26.

McCrae, R. R., & John, O. P. (1992). An introduction to the five-factor model and its applications. *Journal of Personality, 60*, 175–215.

Millon, T. (1987). *Manual for the Millon Clinical Multiaxial Inventory*. Minneapolis, MN: National Computer Systems.

Moskowitz, D. S. (1994). Cross-situational generality and the interpersonal circumplex. *Journal of Personality and Social Psychology, 66*, 921–933.

Mullahy, P. (1970). *Psychoanalysis and interpersonal psychiatry: The contributions of Harry Stack Sullivan*. New York: Science House.

Norman, W. T. (1963). Toward an adequate taxonomy of personality attributes: Replicated factor structure in peer nomination personality ratings. *Journal of Abnormal and Social Psychology, 66*, 574–583.

Norman, W. T. (1967). *2800 personality trait descriptors: Normative operating characteristics for a university population*. Ann Arbor: Department of Psychology, University of Michigan.

Orford, J. (1986). The rules of interpersonal complementarity: Does hostility beget hostility and dominance, submission? *Psychological Review, 93*, 365–377.

Parsons, T., & Bales, R. F. (1955). *Family, socialization and interaction process*. Glencoe, IL: Free Press.

Paul, G. L. (1966). *Insight vs. desensitization in psychotherapy*. Stanford, CA: Stanford University Press.

Peabody, D., & Goldberg, L. R. (1989). Some determinants of factor structures from personality trait-descriptors. *Journal of Personality and Social Psychology, 57*, 552–567.

Pincus, A. L. (1994). The interpersonal circumplex and the interpersonal theory: Perspectives on personality and its pathology. In S. Strack & M. Lorr (Eds.), *Differentiating normal and abnormal personality* (pp. 114–136). New York: Springer.

Pincus, A. L., & Wiggins, J. S. (1990). Interpersonal problems and conceptions of personality disorders. *Journal of Personality Disorders, 4*, 342–352.

Pincus, A. L., & Wiggins, J. S. (1992). An expanded perspective on interpersonal assessment. *Journal of Counseling and Development, 71*, 91–94.

Plutchik, R., & Platman, S. R. (1977). Personality connotations of psychiatric diagnoses: Implications for a similarity model. *Journal of Nervous and Mental Disease, 165*, 418–421.

Random House unabridged dictionary (2nd ed.). (1993). New York: Random House.

Rank, O. (1945). *Will therapy and Truth and reality*. New York: Knopf.

Redfield, R. (1960). How society operates. In H. L. Shapiro (Ed.), *Man, culture, and society* (pp. 345–368). New York: Oxford University Press.

Redfield, R. (1962). The peasant's view of the good life. In M. P. Redfield (Ed.), *Human nature and the study of society: The papers of Robert Redfield* (Vol. 1, pp. 310–326). Chicago: University of Chicago Press.

Rogers, C. R. (1961). *On becoming a person: A therapist's view of psychotherapy.* Boston: Houghton Mifflin.

Rotter, J. B. (1954). *Social learning and clinical psychology.* Englewood Cliffs, NJ: Prentice-Hall.

Runyon, W. McK. (1988). A historical and conceptual background to psychohistory. In W. McK. Runyon (Ed.), *Psychology and historical interpretation* (pp. 3–60). New York: Oxford University Press.

Sadalla, E. K., Kenrick, D. T., & Vershure, B. (1987). Dominance and heterosexual attraction. *Journal of Personality and Social Psychology, 52,* 730–738.

Saucier, G. (1992). Openness versus intellect: Much ado about nothing? *European Journal of Personality, 8,* 273–290.

Schaefer, E. S., & Plutchik, R. (1966). Interrelationships of emotions, traits, and diagnostic constructs. *Psychological Reports, 18,* 399–410.

Snell, W. E., Jr., McDonald, K., & Koch, W. R. (1991). Anger provoking experiences: A multidimensional scaling analysis. *Personality and Individual Differences, 12,* 1095–1104.

Soldz, S., Budman, S., Demby, A., & Merry, J. (1993). Representation of personality disorders in circumplex and five-factor space: Explorations with a clinical sample. *Psychological Assessment, 5,* 41–52.

Spence, J. T. (1985). Gender identity and its implications for the concepts of masculinity and femininity. In T. B. Sonderegger (Ed.), *1984 Nebraska symposium on motivation* (Vol. 32, pp. 59–95). Lincoln: University of Nebraska Press.

Spence, J. T., & Helmreich, R. L. (1978). *Masculinity and femininity: Their psychological dimensions, correlates, and antecedents.* Austin: University of Texas Press.

Steiner, C. M. (1974). *Scripts people live.* New York: Grove Press.

Sullivan, H. S. (1948). The meaning of anxiety in psychiatry and in life. *Psychiatry, 11,* 1–13.

Sullivan, H. S. (1953a). *The interpersonal theory of psychiatry.* New York: Norton.

Sullivan, H. S. (1953b). *Conceptions of modern psychiatry.* New York: Norton.

Sullivan, H. S. (1954). *The psychiatric interview.* New York: Norton.

Sullivan, H. S. (1956). *Clinical studies in psychiatry.* New York: Norton.

Swensen, C. H., Jr. (1973). *Introduction to interpersonal relations.* Glenview, IL: Scott, Foresman.

Taylor, J. A. (1953). A personality scale of manifest anxiety. *Journal of Abnormal and Social Psychology, 48,* 285–290.

Tellegen, A. (1985). Structure of mood and personality and their relevance to assessing anxiety, with an emphasis on self-report. In A. H. Tuma & J.

D. Maser (Eds.), *Anxiety and the anxiety disorders* (pp. 681–706). Hillsdale, NJ: Erlbaum.

Tellegen, A. (1994). *Manual for the Multidimensional Personality Questionnaire.* Minneapolis: University of Minnesota Press.

Tellegen, A., & Atkinson, G. (1974). Openness to absorbing and self-altering experiences. *Journal of Abnormal Psychology, 83,* 268–277.

Tellegen A., & Waller, N. G. (in press). Exploring personality through test construction: Development of the Multidimensional Personality Questionnaire. In S. R. Briggs & J. M. Cheek (Eds.), *Personality measures: Development and evaluation* (Vol. 1). Greenwich, CT: JAI Press.

Tomkins, S. S. (1965). Affect and the psychology of knowledge. In S. S. Tomkins & C. E. Izard (Eds.), *Affect, cognition, and personality: Empirical studies* (pp. 72–97). New York: Springer.

Tracey, T. J., & Rounds, J. B. (1993). Evaluating Holland's and Gati's vocational interest models: A structural meta-analysis. *Psychological Bulletin, 113,* 299–246.

Trapnell, P. D. (1989). *Structural validity in the measurement of Holland's vocational typology: A measure of Holland's types scaled to an explicit circumplex model.* Unpublished master's thesis, University of British Columbia, Vancouver.

Trapnell, P. D. (1992, August). Vocational interests and the facet structure of Factor V. In J. F. Kihlstrom (Chair), *Intellectance and openness in the "Big Five" personality structure.* Symposium at the 100th annual meeting of the American Psychological Association, Washington, DC.

Trapnell, P. D. (1994). Openness versus intellect: A lexical left turn. *European Journal of Personality, 8,* 273–290.

Trapnell, P. D., & Wiggins, J. S. (1990). Extension of the Interpersonal Adjective Scales to include the Big Five dimensions of personality. *Journal of Personality and Social Psychology, 59,* 781–790.

Triandis, H. C. (1990). Cross-cultural studies of individualism and collectivism. In J. J. Berman (Ed.), *1989 Nebraska symposium on motivation: Cross-cultural perspectives* (Vol. 37, pp. 41–133). Lincoln: University of Nebraska Press.

Triandis, H. C. (1995). *Individualism and collectivism.* Boulder, CO: Westview Press.

Triandis, H. C., Bontempo., R., Betancourt, H., Bond, M., Leung, K., Brenes, A., Georgas, J., Hui, C. H., Marin, G., Setiadi, B., Sinha, J. B. P., Verman, J., Spangenberg, J., Touzard, H., & Montmollin, G. (1986). The measurement of the etic aspects of individualism and collectivism across cultures. *Australian Journal of Psychology, 38,* 257–267.

Triandis, H. C., Leung, K., Villareal, M., & Clack, F. L. (1985). Allocentric vs. idiocentric tendencies: Convergent and discriminant validation. *Journal of Research in Personality, 19,* 395–415.

Trivers, R. (1972). Parental investment and sexual selection. In B. Campbell (Ed.), *Sexual selection and the descent of man* (pp. 136–179). Chicago: Aldine-Atherton.

Tupes, E. C., & Christal, R. E. (1992). Recurrent personality factors based on trait ratings. *Journal of Personality, 60,* 225–251. (Original work published 1961)

Turner, J. L., Foa, E. B., & Foa, U. G. (1971). Interpersonal reinforcers: Classification, interrelationship, and some differential properties. *Journal of Personality and Social Psychology, 19,* 168–180.

Watson, D., & Friend, R. (1969). Measurement of social-evaluative anxiety. *Journal of Consulting and Clinical Psychology, 33,* 448–457.

Widiger, T. A., & Frances, A. J. (1994). Toward a dimensional model for the personality disorders. In P. T. Costa, Jr. & T. A. Widiger (Eds.), *Personality disorders and the five-factor model of personality* (pp. 19–39). Washington, DC: American Psychological Association.

Widiger, T. A., & Kelso, K. (1983). Psychodiagnosis of Axis II. *Clinical Psychology Review, 3,* 491–510.

Wiggins, J. S. (1965). Interpersonal Diagnosis of Personality. In O. K. Buros (Ed.), *The sixth mental measurements yearbook* (pp. 451–453). Highland Park, NJ: Gryphon Press.

Wiggins, J. S. (1968). Personality structure. In P. R. Farnsworth (Ed.), *Annual review of psychology* (Vol. 19, pp. 320–322). Palo Alto: Annual Reviews.

Wiggins, J. S. (1973). *Personality and prediction: Principles of personality assessment.* Reading, MA: Addison-Wesley. (Reprinted 1988, Malabar, FL: Krieger)

Wiggins, J. S. (1979). A psychological taxonomy of trait-descriptive terms: The interpersonal domain. *Journal of Personality and Social Psychology, 37,* 295–412.

Wiggins, J. S. (1980). Circumplex models of interpersonal behavior. In L. Wheeler (Ed.), *Review of personality and social psychology* (Vol. 1, pp. 265–293). Beverly Hills, CA: Sage.

Wiggins, J. S. (1982). Circumplex models of interpersonal behavior in clinical psychology. In P. C. Kendall & J. N. Butcher (Eds.), *Handbook of research methods in clinical psychology* (pp. 183–221). New York: Wiley.

Wiggins, J. S. (1984). Cattell's system from the perspective of mainstream personality theory. *Multivariate Behavioral Research, 19,* 176–190.

Wiggins, J. S. (1985). Interpersonal circumplex models: 1948–1983 (Commentary). *Journal of Personality Assessment, 49,* 626–631.

Wiggins, J. S. (1987, August). How interpersonal are the MMPI personality disorder scales? In *Current research in MMPI personality disorder scales.* Seminar at the 95th annual meeting of the American Psychological Association, San Francisco, CA.

Wiggins, J. S. (1991a). Agency and communion as conceptual coordinates for the understanding and measurement of interpersonal behavior. In W. Grove & D. Cicchetti (Eds.), *Thinking clearly about psychology: Essays in honor of Paul E. Meehl* (Vol. 2, pp. 89–113). Minneapolis: University of Minnesota Press.

Wiggins, J. S. (1991b, August). Conceptal and structural considerations in the assessment of interpersonal problems. In L. E. Alden (Chair), *Assessment of interpersonal problems: Implications for treatment and research.* Symposium at the 99th annual meeting of the American Psychological Association, San Francisco, CA.

Wiggins, J. S. (1995). *Interpersonal Adjective Scales: Professional manual.* Odessa, FL: Psychological Assessment Resources.

Wiggins, J. S. (in press). In defense of traits. In R. Hogan, J. A. Johnson, & S. R. Briggs (Eds.), *Handbook of personality psychology.* Orlando, FL: Academic Press.

Wiggins, J. S., & Broughton, R. (1991). A geometric taxonomy of personality scales. *European Journal of Personality, 5,* 343–365.

Wiggins, J. S., Phillips, N., & Trapnell, P. (1989). Circular reasoning about interpersonal behavior: Evidence concerning some untested assumptions underlying diagnostic classification. *Journal of Personality and Social Psychology, 56,* 296–305.

Wiggins, J. S., & Pincus, A. L. (1989). Conceptions of personality disorders and dimensions of personality. *Psychological Assessment, 1,* 305–316.

Wiggins, J. S., & Pincus, A. L. (1992). Personality: Structure and assessment. In M. R. Rosenzweig & L. R. Porter (Eds.), *Annual review of psychology* (Vol. 43, pp. 473–504). Palo Alto, CA: Annual Reviews.

Wiggins, J. S., & Pincus, A. L. (1994). Personality structure and the structure of personality disorders. In P. T. Costa, Jr. & T. A. Widiger (Eds.), *Personality disorders and the five-factor model of personality* (pp. 73–93). Washington, DC: American Psychological Association.

Wiggins, J. S., Steiger, J. H., & Gaelick, L. (1981). Evaluating circumplexity in personality data. *Multivariate Behavioral Research, 16,* 263–289.

Wiggins, J. S., & Trapnell, P. D. (in press). Personality structure: The return of the Big Five. In R. Hogan, J. A. Johnson, & S. R. Briggs (Eds.), *Handbook of personality psychology.* Orlando, FL: Academic Press.

Winter, D. (1973). *The power motive.* New York: Free Press.

CHAPTER FIVE

A Socioanalytic Perspective on the Five-Factor Model

ROBERT HOGAN

The use of adjectives (trait-names)—words such as "energetic," "neat," "prudish," "conscientious," "friendly," "submissive," and so forth—to describe repeated manifestations of personality, has not only proved suitable for ordinary discourse, but is necessary . . . in scientific communications, to describe the recurrent characteristics of a given individual's behavior. But to decide that the representation of every individual as a cluster of outstanding traits is the goal would be tantamount to the abandonment of all hope of understanding personality. Each trait-name stands for a highly abstract attribute of overt, and hence peripheral, activity; and once a number of these attributes have been abstracted from the stream of processes, there is no possibility of reassembling them to form a model of the interrelated dynamic systems which constitute personality. Personality is the architecture of the whole, not a list of adjectives descriptive of those parts or aspects which most impress observers.

—MURRAY AND KLUCKHOHN (1953, p. 11)

Proponents of the five-factor model (FFM) imply that personality can be understood in terms of the five broad traits of adjustment, extraversion, conscientiousness, agreeableness, and a combination of imagination and curiosity. The quote from Henry Murray at the top of this page summarizes—in Victorian prose—my perspective on the FFM. The following describes how I would defend that perspective.

In order fully to understand the FFM, we need to discuss at least four topics; these include (1) a theory of personality; (2) a theory of traits; (3) a theory of measurement; and (4) a theory of the link between personality theory and personality measurement. This chapter is organized in terms of these four topics; it begins with an overview of socioanalytic theory in order to provide a context for discussing traits and trait measurement.

Socioanalytic Theory

I have argued, since I was a graduate student at Berkeley in the mid-1960s, that personality psychology suffers from three generic problems that trivialize the discipline and make progress difficult. The first problem concerns the implicit requirement that we study "theories of the middle range," a notion imported into psychology by way of the sociologist R. K. Merton. In contrast, I believe that the legitimate subject matter of the field is the nature of human nature; the old-timers—Freud, Jung, Adler, McDougall, and Murray—knew this. We seem to have forgotten it, and the field has lost its focus as a result.

The second problem concerns the fact that, under the influence of behaviorism and learning theory, psychology took physics as a model for theory building and self-evaluation. I have always thought that psychology was a branch of biology, not physics—I was a physics major—and that evolutionary theory should be the model for theory building and evaluation. Again, the old timers—Freud, Jung, McDougall, and Murray—knew this.

The third problem concerns the fact that, sometime around World War II, largely stimulated by the development of the Minnesota Multiphasic Personality Inventory (MMPI), personality theory and personality assessment split apart. Today we have theories of personality and we have measurement methods; people who are interested in theory seem uninterested in measurement, and people who are interested in measurement seem uninterested in theory. It is true that Carl Rogers, the theorist, experimented with the Q-sort, and that Raymond Cattell, the psychometrician, wrote about morality and religion, but Rogers's statistical experimentation and Cattell's theoretical musings were relatively uninspired.

Socioanalytic theory tries to deal with these three problems; it proposes a model of human nature that is empirically grounded, that is consistent with evolutionary theory, and that can account for its own database (i.e., the theory can explain its measurement procedures).

McCrae and Costa (Chapter 3, this volume) note that "the FFM is based on a commitment to rigorous quantitative science and an assumption of human rationality" (pp. 58–59). In contrast, socioanalytic theory is based on a commitment to evolutionary theory, naturalistic observation, and the inevitability of human self-deception. Let's see if I can make some sense out of this statement.

Assumptions

Socioanalytic theory attempts to combine the most valid insights of Freud and psychoanalysis (Bowlby, 1980) with the most valid insights of G. H. Mead and role theory (Goffman, 1958; Sarbin, 1954)—see also Eibl-Eibesfeldt (1989). The essential features of the model can be summarized in terms of five propositions.

1. Human nature/personality is best understood in the context of human evolution; we are products of the original conditions of evolutionary adaptation.

2. People evolved as group-living, culture-using animals; people always live in groups, every group has a status hierarchy, and the rules for living within that hierarchy are part of culture.

3. People are primarily motivated by—what they do each day is determined by—a small number of unconscious biological needs. Our evolutionary history suggests that people need social acceptance—which facilitates group living and enhances individual survival—and status—which confers on the persons who have it preferential opportunities for reproductive success; that is, the more acceptance and status a person enjoys, the more likely it is that that person will be able successfully to reproduce, and reproductive fitness is the bottom line in evolutionary theory.

4. People are in a sense compelled to interact with one another, and at a deep level, their interactions largely concern negotiating for status and acceptance—this is "the politics of everyday life." Social interaction is, ultimately, an exchange process, and that which is exchanged is status and acceptance (Wiggins, 1980).

5. There is an inherent tension in social life, because actions that enhance status tend to diminish acceptance, and actions that increase acceptance tend to reduce status; that is, success often comes at the expense of another person or group—when one wins, another loses—and this creates rivalries; acceptance is normally achieved by con-

forming to the rules of another person's game (cf. Hogan & Henley, 1969)—and conformity diminishes opportunites for success.

Personality

MacKinnon (1944) notes that the word "personality" in English has two meanings in German: *personlichkeit*, the impression a person gives off; and *personalitat*, the inner aspects of the self. Drawing on this teutonic lexical insight, socioanalytic theory distinguishes between personality from the perspective of the observer and from the perspective of the actor. Personality from the observer's perspective consists of our views of the distinctive features of another person's behavior, and these distinctive features are reflected in that person's reputation. Trait words describe reputations; they are, therefore, inherently evaluative, because reputations reflect the degree of status and social acceptance a person enjoys in his or her community.

Allport (1937) dismissed reputations as a "peripheral" issue in personality psychology—he believed personality psychology was about intrapsychic rather than interpersonal processes. But a person's reputation is a central part of his or her personality; much of what people do each day involves protecting their reputations—and it really matters. On July 20, 1993, Vincent W. Foster, Jr., the Deputy White House Counsel, drove to a park overlooking the Potomac River and shot himself. Official Washington was shocked that a man with so much talent and career potential would do such a thing.

Foster was the commencement speaker at the University of Arkansas law school graduation in 1993; the *New York Times* reports that he told the class: "Dents to the reputation in the legal profession are irreparable." During the next few weeks, he was badly criticized in the editorial section of the *Wall Street Journal*, the Bible of his former clients in Little Rock. The *New York Times* (August 22, 1993) suggested that Mr. Foster killed himself because he thought his reputation among his Arkansas friends and business associates had been ruined by forces outside his control. My point is that, if people will kill over a threat to their reputations, then reputations are not trivial—even from an intrapsychic perspective.

Personality from the observer's perspective can be assessed with reasonable reliability (cf. Funder & Sneed, 1993), and these assessments can be used to forecast future behavior—a person who has a reputation for being clever will sometimes be witty, and a person with a reputation as a thief will sometimes steal.

Personality from the perspective of the actor concerns the structures inside a person that cause or explain his or her reputation.
Knowledge regarding personality from the actor's perspective has
not advanced as rapidly as knowledge about personality from the
observer's perspective, because it must be studied indirectly. Consider, for example, a lugubrious 45-year-old man who claims that he
is morose because he was rejected by his mother, who has been dead
for 30 years. We can in principle verify this claim, but not with the
same reliability that we can verify statements about his reputation.
Despite the problems associated with studying personality from the
actor's perspective, two of its components seem relatively well established: (1) genetically based temperaments (A. H. Buss & Plomin,
1975); and (2) the story that an actor typically tells about him- or
herself (McAdams, 1993), which I refer to as an idealized self-image
or identity.

Interaction

As noted earlier, people are by nature compelled to interact; as
Goffman (1958) observed, interaction is "where the action is." People
need attention and acceptance in a structured format, and these
needs are typically satisfied during interaction. During interaction,
respect and acceptance are exchanged on the basis of a person's
preexisting status and his or her performance during the interaction.
Thus, at social gatherings, high status people will be the focus of the
exchange process. Le Carré (1992) captures this point nicely in the
following scene, which introduces his most recent villain:

> As his boat now mastered the harbor, so . . . Mr. Richard Onslow
> Roper mastered the round table, the terrace, and the restaurant.
> Unlike his boat he was not dressed for spectacle. . . . Neverthe-
> less, he commanded. By the stillness of his patrician head. By the
> speed of his smile and the intelligence of his expression. By the
> attention lavished on him by his audience, whether he spoke or
> listened. By the way everything around the table, from the dishes
> to the bottles . . . to the faces of the children, seemed to be
> ranged toward him or away from him. (p. 165)

What do we need in order to have an interaction? Every interaction has the same underlying structure. There will be an agenda—a
project, pretext, or theme around which the interaction is organized—and there will be roles or parts to play during the interaction.

Everyday life consists of moving from one interaction sequence to another, and each interaction will have its own agenda and corresponding roles. We need to interact and, outside of our roles, we have little to say to one another.

Roles

Roles are the parts we play during interaction, and every interaction, as noted earlier, requires that roles be available. Very formal interactions—wedding ceremonies—are tightly scripted, which means that the roles are formal, and there will be little variation in how they are played, regardless of who is in them. Informal interactions—conversations in a bar—are loosely scripted and the part we play is our own—our identities are the generalized roles that we carry with us from interaction to interaction.

Formal roles are rooted in the history of a culture. Informal roles or identities are rooted in the history of each person's development. Identities begin with temperament—being shy will constrain a person's interactional style in certain ways. But identities are largely shaped by a person's efforts to negotiate acceptance and status during interactions from childhood to early adulthood. Unlike adolescents, adults tend not to be self-conscious about their identities.

Identities—personality from the actor's perspective—translate into reputations—personality from the observer's perspective—because each identity dictates a certain self-presentational style. Thus the amount of status and acceptance that a person enjoys is directly related to his or her indentity.

Why are there individual differences in status and social acceptance? Why doesn't everyone simply adopt an identity that will maximize his or her social rewards? This is where socioanalytic theory departs company from much of modern psychology. People are not rational. Adults are typically unaware of the identities that guide their social behavior, and they are often careless about or indifferent to the manner in which others react to them. In addition, some people are more attentive to these processes than others—extraverts versus introverts; some occupations require more attention to these processes than others—actors versus accountants; some people may be inherently more socially skilled than others—John Kennedy versus Richard Nixon; and there are accidents of birth. For example, children growing up on farms are typically taught to be frank and candid and not to allow others to bully or intimidate them. This translates into an indentity and a self-presentational style that is seriously maladaptive in modern corporate America, where success depends on hypocricy and flattery (sometimes called diplomacy) and the ability to "go with the flow."

Finally, everybody has to be somebody; everybody has to have an identity in order to interact with others and take part in the social process. Identities are based on the models that are available in a person's immediate social environment. Children of poverty, for example, have only a limited range of models on which to draw, and as a result, they often construct self-defeating identities. All of this, again, takes place outside of immediate consciousness.

Even those persons who claim only "to be themselves" must put on a careful act in order to let others know that they are, in fact, being themselves (Schlenker & Weigold, 1990). People choose their activities and interactions as part of the process of self-presentation. Helping the poor supports an altruistic identity; driving a motorcycle supports a daring identity; publishing scholarly articles supports an intellectual identity. No matter what a person's intentions may be during an interaction, others will assume that what that person is doing is intended to tell others about how he or she would like to be regarded. Finally, all of these processes are at work, even when the interaction is a psychological experiment or an assessment center exercise.

Agendas

During social interaction, people's behavior is constrained by the agenda for the interaction. Moreover, just as people can play more than one role simultaneously, more than one agenda can operate during an interaction—for example, whatever else is going on, each person will, at some level, be trying not to lose status or acceptance. Nonetheless, it would be useful to have a taxonomy of agendas.

Here is where Holland's (1985) model of people and occupations is very helpful. Hogan, Raza, and Driskell (1988) show that military teams can be classified quite reliably into Holland-types on the basis of their primary tasks—most of which are a combination of Realistic and Conventional activities. Similarly, we should be able to classify interactions on the basis of their primary tasks. This leads me to believe that there are probably six major agendas, individually or in combination, for interactions. We can get together and fix something (Realistic), analyze something (Investigative), entertain someone (Artistic), help someone (Social), persuade and manipulate someone (Enterprising), or regulate something (Conventional).

Finally, Holland and his colleagues have provided overwhelming evidence that people prefer activities and interactions that are consistent with their identities, and they dislike activities and interactions that are discordant with their identities. So, for example, Artistic people prefer and enjoy Artistic tasks and interactions and dislike Conventional tasks and interactions.

The Socioanalytic Theory of Traits

Traits are the most common unit of analysis in personality psychology. Various writers (e.g., McCrae & Costa, Chapter 3, this volume) argue that traits are the correct or real units of analysis in personality research, but not everyone agrees with this judgment. Part of the problem is that there is a fair amount of confusion surrounding the seemingly simple notion of a trait.

The primary referent for the trait concept is a consistent pattern of thoughts, feelings, and actions. These consistent patterns might be our own or they might be reported by others; either way, trait words refer to consistencies in the actions and experiences of people.

So far, so good. The issue begins to get messy, however, when we ask about the function of trait terms: What are they used for and what do they do for us? Some writers (e.g., D. M. Buss & Craik, 1983a) argue that trait words describe the consistencies that we see in the behavior of others; thus, we use trait terms for the purpose of description, communication, and classification (e.g., to say that Jones is an aggressive person means that Jones often acts in ways that others regard as aggressive, but the reason he does so is a matter for further investigation). Using traits for description and classification leads to some very useful results (cf. D. M. Buss & Craik, 1983b), but it is a pretheoretical exercise; description and classification do not require that we take a position on the nature of traits per se.

Other writers believe that trait words not only *describe* consistencies in people's actions, but also they *explain* them as well. Putting the matter somewhat crudely, the argument seems to be that beneath a pattern of, for example, aggressive behavior is a trait for aggressiveness. Here the word trait is a shorthand term for a hypothesized underlying neurological, hormonal, or biochemical construct; it might be a genetic predisposition toward hyperactivity and social insensitivity, it might be an active region in the hippocampus, or it might be a pervasive mood state. The point, however, is that this notion of a trait assumes three things: (1) the existence of a detectable pattern of consistent feelings and behavior; (2) the existence of an underlying neurobiological structure that causes the feelings and behavior; and (3) the ability to map, on a point-for-point basis, the feelings and behavior onto their cause.

This view of traits originates, at least in American psychology, with Gordon Allport (1937). Allport's discussion is sophisticated (cf. Zuroff, 1986). For example, he distinguishes between the traits that psychologists use to describe other people and the traits that people use to describe themselves; the first are the scales on standard personality inventories; the second come from individual interviews. He also distinguishes between traits as stylistic consistencies in behavior, and traits as underlying "neuropsychic structures." After drawing all these distinctions, Allport then claims that the "real units of analysis in personality psychology" are individual traits that originate in underlying neurophysiological structures.

The Allportian view is popular in modern psychology; prominent advocates include McCrae and Costa (Chapter 3, this volume), Funder (1991), and Tellegen (1991). This perspective is aligned with the traditional scientific worldview. It is reductionist—surface level or behavioral regularities are traced to underlying biological and physiological mechanisms. And it is positivistic—although the nature of the underlying mechanisms is obscure and the means to link personality test scores to the underlying mechanisms doesn't exist, the advocates of this position have faith that the links will be found. The original meaning of positivism concerned faith in the possibility of scientific progress.

The data that support this position come from two sources. The first is consistencies in a person's responses to questionnaire items; the second is consistencies in a person's behavior as reported or observed by others. When responses to questionnaire items cluster together, or when consistencies are observed in the behavior of another person, one can hypothesize that the consistencies are caused by particular neurological structures; this hypothesis is supported only in a probabilistic sense: "Unfortunately, a method to assess the neural basis of personality is not yet in sight. The presence of a trait can only be inferred on the basis of overt behavior" (Funder, 1991, p. 32). In my view, that inference is too much of a stretch.

Traits refer to observed consistencies in behavior. From the perspective of socioanalytic theory, traits are the terms that observers use to describe actors. Although actors can describe themselves using trait terms when they are asked, this is not how they would normally describe themselves. Trait words are typically the linguistic tools of observers; they are the cognitive categories that observers use to encode the distinctive features of an actor's behavior. Reputations, therefore, are encoded in trait words, and this is a very useful fact. Reputations are stable, reputations predict future behavior, people care deeply about their reputations, and, because reputations are publicly observable, statements about reputations can be verified.

I believe that trait words originate in the perceptual categories of observers (see also D. M. Buss & Craik, 1983a); we describe, remember, and evaluate the behavior of others using trait terms. What, from this perspective, is inside actors that accounts for the stable features of their behavior that we observe? We really don't know, although it is an interesting topic on which to speculate.

Perhaps an example would illustrate the difference in the conventional and socioanalytic perspectives on traits. Consider the concept of "shyness"; it is a common phenomenon, and a number of excellent measures of the shyness construct have been developed (Jones, Cheek, & Briggs, 1986). In the standard theory of traits, shy people are believed to have a particular genetic constitution that makes them socially awkward, reluctant to talk to strangers, and prone to feeling distressed in unfamiliar social circumstances. "Shyness" refers to a distinctive pattern of social behavior and to an underlying genetic makeup.

From a socioanalytic perspective, being socially diffident and reluctant to talk to strangers can also be (perhaps unconsciously) an interpersonal strategy. It is easy to argue, based on knowledge of our evolutionary history, that talking to strangers has usually been dangerous, and that we will normally find it stressful. In polite society, however, enduring that stress is part of the price of admission to social interaction. Certain people may be unwilling to pay the price and excuse themselves by being "shy." By being known as shy, a person can avoid many of the less pleasant burdens of social life, such as making small talk with dull people at receptions and cocktail parties. Moreover, when shy people put the burden for sustaining an interaction on others, they can often control an interaction as the others attempt to draw them out—following the principle that he or she who is least interested in sustaining an interaction will control it. Thus, there are a number of advantages to being shy, and these advantages may outweigh the disadvantages—whatever they may be.

As suggested earlier, observers code the characteristic features of another person's social behavior in terms of trait words, and the composite of agreed upon trait words used to describe a person becomes that person's reputation. Reputations are stable, enduring, and can be used to forecast future behavior. But the most interesting feature of reputations for a personality psychologist is that they have a well-defined structure, and this, I believe, is what the five-factor model (FFM) is all about. The FFM *primarily* concerns the structure of observer ratings (cf. Paunonen, 1993). There have been demonstrations that self-descriptions can be organized in terms of the FFM, but this is, I believe, an artifact of the factoring process (cf. Block, 1995); that is, almost any analysis can be constrained to a five-factor solution, but the natural structure of self-ratings is always more complex than five factors.

Everyone has a reputation, and every reputation can be profiled in terms of the FFM. Why is this? Recall that people evolved as group-living animals. Recall also that each person is motivated to seek status and social acceptance, and that these resources come from other people—they are what is exchanged during interactions (Wiggins, 1980). The FFM contains the categories that people use to evaluate one another; through the vehicle of reputation, these categories reveal the amount of status and acceptance that a person has been granted, and that he or she can normally expect to receive. A "reputation," defined in terms of the FFM, is an index of how well a person is doing in the game of life. Because the game, at a deep level, concerns reproductive success, it is ultimately quite serious.

People evolved as group-living animals. Thus, each person in a group was a potential contributor to or detractor from the success of his or her group vis-a-vis the other groups with which it was in competition. In this context, reputations, as encoded in the FFM, may have forecast a person's utility in the economy of his or her group. For example, the Adjustment dimension concerns how well a person will perform under pressure and how emotionally stable he or she is on a day-to-day basis. The Sociability/Ambition dimension concerns leadership potential. The Prudence dimension concerns trustworthiness and dependability. The Likability dimension concerns how much others enjoy a person's company. The Intellectance dimension concerns the degree to which a person will be a resource for solving technical problems confronting the group—as Odysseus, the inventor of the Trojan Horse and, therefore, the ultimate conqueror of Troy, said when the mighty Achilles went down, "So much for Greek courage, now for Greek cunning."

In summary, from a socioanalytic perspective, the dimensions of the FFM resemble Jungian archetypes; they are innate categories of human perception used to evaluate the potential contribution of others to the success of one's family, tribe, corporation, or combat unit. The FFM is the property of observers, and it is used to predict and evaluate the behavior of others. Ultimately, evaluations framed in terms of the FFM tell us about an actor's standing in his or her social community. Smart players in the game of life know that they are being evaluated, they know what the categories of evaluation are, and they try to control how they are evaluated. Other players seem not to understand—or perhaps care about—the evaluation process.

A Socioanalytic Theory of Measurement

The standard view of personality measurement is that responses to items on a personality measure are "self-reports." This view is consistent with Allport's notion that if you want to know why a person acts in a particular way, you need only ask, and the person will tell you. Thus, so the argument goes, we can ask people if they are typically dominant, aggressive, anxious, or self-confident, and they can tell us. We can then use their responses to evaluate the degree to which they have dominant, aggressive, anxious, or self-confident traits.

The presumed dynamics of this self-report process seem to be as follows: We interact with others, and they respond to us; we store their reactions somewhere in our memories. Over time we reflect on how others have reacted to us. From these reflections, we build up views of ourselves—for example, "When I think about how others react to me, I must conclude that I am (lazy, stupid, impulsive, etc.) disposed to act in certain characteristic ways."

On a later occasion, in response to an item on a questionnaire such as "I think I am somewhat lazy," we call up our views of ourselves in instances in which laziness might have been involved, we compare our internal self-view with the item, and we endorse the item one way or another.

This perspective is supported by the frequent finding that the most valid items on personality scales are also the items with the greatest face validity—or so it seems after the items have been validated. For example, the best item on Hogan's (1969) Empathy scale is "I have little trouble putting myself in another person's shoes." The role taking tendencies implicit in this item are at the core of Hogan's notion of empathy; nonetheless, Hogan could not say, prior to conducting the analyses, that that item would be the best one on the scale. Thus, the finding that the most face-valid items are the most empirically valid is a judgment that is always made after the fact.

There is a major problem with the self-report view of personality measurement. The problem concerns the fact that memory doesn't work the way the model assumes it does. Memory is not like a videotape that we call up and play back when we need it. Modern research (Neisser & Winograd, 1988) suggests that we construct our memories. Moreover, we often construct them in self-serving ways. Memories are our theories about how we were, and they are often simply wrong. Memories are not necessarily veridical; rather than being reliable empirical records about ourselves, they are often the products of the revisionist tendencies that Nietzsche and Freud described so well.

Following Goffman (1958), Sarbin (1954), and others, socioanalytic theory assumes that during social interaction, people, at some level, are concerned with controlling—as far as it is possible to do so—the manner in which others react to them. More specifically, people have idealized views of themselves—for example, as someone who is dangerous when provoked, as someone who can get this country moving again, as someone who is competent to treat your medical complaint—and during social interaction, they are motivated to convince others that these idealized views are true.

This perspective also assumes that the same processes that guide social interaction guide people's responses to items on personality questionnaires. Item endorsements, therefore, are self-presentations, not self-reports. Moreover, consistencies in the pattern of a person's item endorsements reflect consistent styles of self-presentation rather than underlying traits. And finally, this position argues that the process of self-presentation—during social interaction or in response to questionnaire items—is not necessarily or even routinely conscious. Rather, the manner in which we present ourselves and the image that we try to maintain are often unconscious, or at least outside of awareness.

Conventional trait theory assumes a point-for-point correspondence between item endorsements and underlying traits; people who endorse items referring to dominant behavior are expected to see themselves as dominant and perhaps to be disposed on occasion to behave in a dominant fashion. The socioanalytic perspective, however, makes no such assumption about the link between item endorsements and other behavior. Rather, in agreement with Meehl (1948), this perspective regards an item endorsement as an interesting behavior whose nontest meaning must be discovered empirically. An item endorsement is a symbolic act, not a self-report, and in order to determine what it means, one must do some research.

The Link between Theory and Measurement

As noted in the beginning of this chapter, socioanalytic theory attempts to combine the valid insights of psychoanalysis and symbolic interactionism. What might these insights be? From Freud we learn that there is an instinctual core to human nature—based on our evolutionary heritage—and that these core instincts move in opposing directions, so that ambivalence is an essential part of the human condition. From George Herbert Mead we learn that people are fundamentally oriented toward social interaction, that psychological processes arise in the context of interaction, and that these processes are best understood in these terms. From Freud and Mead we learn that social behavior is symbolic, that social action is a text to be interpreted. Nothing is as it is, every action is laden with meaning, no act is capable of merely being itself. In the to and fro of everyday social encounter, concrete-minded people who take others' words and actions at face value put themselves at a serious disadvantage— and it doesn't matter if they are dealing with criminals, lunatics, politicians, or behaviorists. Personality psychologists in particular can't afford to make this mistake.

Finally, from Freud we learn that we are typically unaware of the meanings of our actions, that these meanings may be unattractive, and that we would be well advised to maintain a watchful, detached, and even wary attitude toward our impulses. Analysts and therapists spend much of their time unraveling the repetitive, automatic, and self-destructive behaviors that their clients believe are rational and well meaning.

This is the context in terms of which we should understand people's responses to items on personality questionnaires. The tendency in modern psychology is to take these responses at face value—people know themselves and, if so inclined, can tell you what they know. This is a pretheoretical view of item responses, and it has at least three problems.

First, the modern view takes item responses as self-reports, as true accounts of the person's motives, attitudes, goals, and typical ways of treating others. At the least, this begs the question of whether, in an individual case, these accounts are in fact true; at worst, it ignores the problem of self-deception.

Second, the modern view assumes that the link between the theory and its measurement base is systematic and straightforward. This view assumes that scale scores (scores on personality questionnaires) reflect underlying traits, which are neurological entities. Traits are projected into scale scores through a person's responses to the items on the questionnaire. Thus, scale scores measure the degree to which traits penetrate into self-awareness. This assumption ignores the symbolic nature of social interaction. Responding to an item is as much a social act as responding to a question from your mother, and its meaning should be understood in terms of the actor's typical interpersonal goals rather than a hypothesized and unobservable neuropsychic entity.

Finally, the modern view assumes a Platonist theory of meaning. As the reader will recall, Plato argued that the meaning of an object was given by its reference to an abstract and ideal form that exists in another, nontemporal, nonspatial universe; a particular chair should be understood by comparing it to an abstract concept of "chairness." Similarly, in the modern view, a scale score refers to an abstract entity that exists, not in a nontemporal, nonspatial universe, but inside the individual; the meaning of personalty scale scores is given by what the scores refer to—namely entities inside the person.

Socioanalytic theory takes a different view of the nature and meaning of personality scale scores. The model comes from Wittgenstein's (1953) discussion, in which he argues that the meaning of something is given by how it is used rather than by the abstract entity to which it refers. Gough (1968, p. 56; 1987, pp. 3–4; 1989, pp. 69–72) has argued for years that the California Psychological Inventory is not designed to measure traits but to forecast performance. I believe Gough is exactly right; the meaning of a scale score should be determined empirically and depends on what it predicts rather than on the entities to which it refers. This approach puts the issue of validity at the center of any discussion of personality assessment. We will never know how well a scale score captures the essence of an underlying hypothetical trait, but we can determine the fit between a person's score on a measure and how he or she is described by others.

Finally, then, I would note the correspondence between the viewpoint presented here and the one that Murray set forth in 1953, as seen in the opening quote for this chapter. Traits are a useful means for communicating information about others, but the traits themselves are only surface indicators of underlying processes and themes.

Acknowledgments

I thank Alan Elms, Harrison Gough, Allan Harkness, Aaron Pincus, and Jerry Wiggins for their helpful comments on an earlier version of this chapter.

References

Allport, G. W. (1937). *Personality: A psychological interpretation.* New York: Holt.

Block, J. (1995). A contrarian view of the five-factor approach to personality description. *Psychological Bulletin, 117,* 187–215.

Bowlby, J. (1980). *Attachment and loss.* New York: Basic Books.

Buss, A. H., & Plomin, R. (1975). *A temperament theory of personality.* New York: Wiley.

Buss, D. M., & Craik, K. H. (1983a). Act prediction and the conceptual analysis of personality scales. *Journal of Personality and Social Psychology, 45,* 1081–1095.

Buss, D. M., & Craik, K. H. (1983b). The act frequency approach to personality. *Psychological Review, 90,* 105–126.

Eibl-Eibesfeldt, I. (1989). *Human ethology.* New York: Aldine.

Funder, D. C. (1991). Global traits: A neo-Allportian approach to personality. *Psychological Science, 2,* 31–39.

Funder, D. C., & Sneed, C. D. (1993). Behavioral manifestations of personality: An ecological approach to judgmental accuracy. *Journal of Personality and Social Psychology, 64,* 479–490.

Goffman, E. (1958). *The presentation of self in everyday life.* New York: Doubleday.

Gough, H. G. (1968). An interpreter's syllabus for the California Psychological Inventory. In P. McReynolds (Ed.), *Advances in psychological assessment* (Vol. 1, pp. 55–79). Palo Alto, CA: Science & Behavior Books.

Gough, H. G. (1987). *Manual for the California Psychological Inventory.* Palo Alto, CA: Consulting Psychologists Press.

Gough, H. G. (1989). The California psychological inventory. In C. S. Newmark (Ed.), *Major psychological assessment instruments* (Vol. 2, pp. 67–98). Boston: Allyn & Bacon.

Hogan, R. (1969). Development of an empathy scale. *Journal of Consulting and Clinical Psychology, 33,* 307–316.

Hogan, R., & Henley, N. (1969). Nomotics: The science of human rule systems. *American Psychological Association Proceedings,* pp. 443–444.

Hogan, R., Raza, S., & Driskell, J. E (1988). Personality, team performance, and organizational context. In P. Whitney & R. B. Ocsman (Eds.), *Psychology and productivity* (pp. 93–104). New York: Plenum Press.

Holland, J. L. (1985). *Making vocational choices: A theory of personalities and work environments* (2nd ed.). Englewood Cliffs, NJ: Prentice-Hall.

Jones, W. H., Cheek, J. M., & Briggs, S. R. (Eds.). (1986). *Shyness: Perspectives on research and treatment.* New York: Plenum Press.

Le Carré, J. (1993). *The night manager.* New York: Knopf.

MacKinnon, D. W. (1944). The structure of personality. In J. McV. Hunt (Ed.) *Personality and the behavior disorders* (Vol. 1, pp. 4–43) New York: Ronald Press.

McAdams, D. P. (1993). *Stories we live by.* New York: Morrow.

Meehl, P. E. (1948). The "dynamics" of structured personality tests. *Journal of Clinical Psychology, 1,* 296–303.

Murray, H. A. & Kluckhohn, C. (1953). Outline of a conception of personality. In H. A. Murray & C. Kluckhohn (Eds.), *Personality in nature, society, and culture* (2nd ed., pp. 3–32). New York: Knopf.

Neisser, U., & Winograd, E. (1988). *Remembering reconsidered.* Cambridge, UK: Cambridge University Press.

Paunonen, S. V. (1993, August). *Sense, nonsense, and the Big Five factors of personality.* Paper presented at the annual meeting of the American Psychological Association, Toronto, Canada.

Sarbin, T. R. (1954). Role theory. In G. Lindzey (Ed.), *Handbook of social psychology.* (Vol. 1, pp. 223–258). Cambridge, MA.: Addison-Wesley.

Schlenker, B.R., & Weigold, M. F. (1990). Self-consciousness and self-presentation: Being autonomous versus appearing autonomous. *Journal of Personality and Social Psychology, 59,* 820–828.

Tellegen, A. (1991). Personality traits: Issues of definition, evidence, and assessment. In D. Cicchetti & W. Grove (Eds.), *Thinking clearly about psychology: Essays in honor of Paul Everett Meehl* (Vol. 2, pp. 10–35). Minneapolis: University of Minnesota Press.

Wiggins, J. S. (1980). Circumplex models of interpersonal behavior. In L. Wheeler (Ed.), *Review of personality and social psychology* (Vol. 1, pp. 265–294). Beverly Hills, CA: Sage.

Wittgenstein, L. (1953) *Philosophical investigations.* Oxford: Blackwell.

Zuroff, D. C. (1986). Was Gordon Allport a trait theorist? *Journal of Personality and Social Psychology, 51,* 993–100.

CHAPTER SIX

Social Adaptation
and Five Major Factors
of Personality

DAVID M. BUSS

Individuals differ in a number of ways that we tend to notice and talk about. Some tend to be conciliatory, others pugnacious. Some are modest, others bombastic. Some impose their will on the group, others accept the structure provided. According to the lexical hypothesis, the differences that are noticed and talked about tend to become encoded within the natural language as trait terms such as aggressive, agreeable, arrogant, dominant, and submissive, and enter into everyday usage in our communications with others (Norman, 1963).

Individuals also differ in an infinite number of ways that either go unnoticed or are not sufficiently noteworthy to warrant much discussion. Some individuals have belly buttons turned in, others have belly buttons turned out. Some lead with their left foot, others with their right. One key function of personality theory is to identify the *most important* ways in which individuals differ from among the infinite dimensions of possible difference (Goldberg, 1972; Wiggins, 1979).

Within the past decade, personality researchers, using a variety of different theoretical perspectives, have advanced variants of what has become known as the five-factor model—Surgency, Agreeableness, Conscientiousness, Emotional Stability, and Intellect–Openness (Norman, 1963; Goldberg, 1981, 1992; John, 1990; McCrae & Costa, Chapter 3, this volume; Hofstee, De Raad, & Goldberg, 1992; Hogan, 1983 and Chapter 5, this volume; Wiggins & Trapnell, in press).

Theoretical positions on the model include the lexical perspective (Norman, 1963; Goldberg, 1981), the social-exchange perspective (Wiggins, 1979, 1991), and the socioanalytic perspective (Hogan, 1983 and Chapter 5, this volume).

The five-factor model has been criticized on theoretical and empirical grounds (e.g., Block, 1995; Waller & Ben-Porath, 1987). Some of these criticisms call into question the comprehensiveness and precision of the five-factor model. Nonetheless, the model's emergence from and endorsement by personality researchers using different theoretical orientations, its documented empirical links with many major personality inventories and instruments (McCrae & Costa, Chapter 3, this volume), its replicability across different populations and data sources (McCrae & John, 1992), and its links with important interpersonal transactions such as conflict and manipulation (Buss, 1992)—all suggest that the dimensions of individual differences captured by the five-factor model cannot be easily dismissed and deserve serious theoretical attention.

The goal of this chapter is to present an *evolutionary psychological perspective* on the five-factor model of individual differences (see also Buss, 1991b). First, I describe the basic theoretical assumptions of the evolutionary psychology perspective. Second, I offer two primary ways within which individual differences become important: (1) in creating adaptive problems for people (*strategic interference*), and (2) in solving adaptive problems (*strategic facilitation*). Finally, I offer empirical illustrations of social adaptive problems that highlight the potential utility of the evolutionary psychological perspective on the five factors.

Humans as Problem Solvers

From an evolutionary perspective, humans can be considered to be complex collections of integrated mechanisms designed by natural and sexual selection to solve problems. Consider the human body. Our bodies contain many specialized mechanisms designed to solve particular problems. Our livers solve the problem of filtering toxins that can be detrimental to survival. Our callus-producing mechanisms solve the problem of damage to the skin due to repeated friction. Our sweat glands solve the problem of thermal regulation. Our taste preferences solve the problem of selecting substances to ingest (ripe berries, tubers, meat; but not twigs, pebbles, or feces).

Each one of the dozens of mechanisms within our bodies is designed to solve a specific adaptive problem.

There are two key points to this body analogy. First, identifying the *function* of a mechanism is essential to understanding its nature, its design features, the contexts that activate it, and its reason for existing at all. In earlier generations, tonsils were routinely removed when they became infected. Now that we know the function of tonsils in disease prevention, they are rarely removed. Major advances in the life sciences often hinge on identifying function.

Second, there is no other coherent and nonarbitrary way of parsing the human body other than by function. We consider the eyes and the nose to be separate anatomical entities, even though they are close together spatially, because we recognize that the eyes and the nose are designed—each with their own distinctive features—to solve somewhat different adaptive problems. Furthermore, each of these adaptations has its own special design features that are exquisitely tailored to perform the function for which it was designed. The use of nonfunctional criteria for parsing the human body—such as spatial proximity—would result in an incoherent and largely arbitrary segmenting. In short, identifying function is essential for understanding the workings of the human body and provides the only nonarbitrary means for carving the body at its natural joints.

Evolutionary psychologists believe that the same logic applies to the human mind. Just as the body is functionally designed, the mind is functionally designed. Just as the body contains many mechanisms, the mind contains many mechanisms. Just as the mechanisms of the body solve adaptive problems, the mechanisms of the mind solve adaptive problems. Just as identifying adaptive function provides a nonarbitrary means of carving the body at its natural joints, identifying adaptive function provides a nonarbitrary means for carving the mind at its natural joints.

Social Adaptive Problems

Although many of the adaptive problems already noted, such as thermal regulation, protecting the structures beneath the skin, and filtering toxins, are properly described as "survival problems," many adaptive problems do not concern survival. Indeed, evolution operates by differential *reproductive* success by virtue of differences in design features; survival is only important inasmuch as it is typically a requirement for reproduction.

Reproductive problems are heavily saturated with social content. Obvious ones include selecting a mate, attracting a mate, copulating, fending off rivals, and raising children. The fact that humans live in groups and all groups contain social hierarchies (Hogan, 1983, Chapter 5, this volume) creates particular social adaptive problems for humans. Reproductively relevant resources such as food, territory, and desirable mates, for example, typically flow to those higher in the social hierarchy and trickle down only slowly to those at the bottom. Therefore, an evolutionary psychologist expects that selection over time would produce specific psychological mechanisms in humans designed to solve the problems of negotiating and scaling hierarchies, dealing with those higher, lower, and equivalently placed in the hierarchy, and preventing skids or slides in status (Stone, 1989; Kyl-Heku & Buss, under review).

Just as specific food preferences solve the survival problem of consumption, specific mate preferences solve the reproductive problem of consummation. Just as our arteries and veins constrict in the cold to prevent the loss of body heat, our social strategies operate in times of hierarchical instability to prevent the loss of status. Because many of the adaptive problems of reproduction in group-living species are inherently social in nature, evolutionary psychologists anticipate that many of our psychological mechanisms are designed to solve social problems.

Individual Differences Are Crucial
for Solving Social Adaptive Problems

All cars have four wheels, an engine, a set of brakes, and a steering device. These are components of "car nature." All humans have two legs, a heart, opposable thumbs, and a relatively hairless body surface (compared with other primates). These are components of "human nature." Just as cars differ in their wheel base, torque, and steering devices, the components that comprise human nature also vary.

When an engineer designs a car, both the "car nature" and differences in components must be considered in great detail. When choosing a car to purchase, however, the basic components of "car nature" become irrelevant because all cars possess them. Rather, the *differences* among the cars become critical for selection—whether the car is large or small, powerful or weak, economical on gas or a guzzler, and whether it will inflict many costs through unreliability or few costs by maintaining resiliency through bumpy roads and bitter winters.

In the same manner, when we face social adaptive problems such as selecting a mate, it would be preposterous to use "having an opposable thumb" or "two-leggedness" as key selection criteria since, with rare exception, all potential mates have these attributes. Despite the fact that having an opposable thumb is a remarkably important part of human nature, a woman seeking a mate does not think: "Wow, I really find him attractive—he has an opposable thumb!" Constants do not count in decisions of selection. Just as in selecting a car, the differences among individuals loom large.

As an illustration, consider the various social selections we make in everyday life, such as mate selection and leader selection. When we cast our ballots for a president on election day, the fact that both candidates have used their species-typical ability to acquire a language is irrelevant. As in selecting a car, it is the differences that are crucial. Which politician has greater oratory skills, however, may be highly relevant, as will the questions: Which politician is more intelligent and insightful? Which has the surgency to lead us into the uncertainties of the 21st century? Which is more honest? Which shares my values? Which has the international clout to forge alliances with other countries? These differences are all critical to solving the problem of selecting a leader.

Consider a somewhat different type of selection—mate selection. The fact that two potential mates share bipedal locomotion is irrelevant to the selection. Again, it is the differences that become critical. Who is more intelligent? Which is more physically attractive? Who has a more exciting personality? Which shares my values? Who is more honest? Who has a better sense of humor? Who is better in bed? Who is more likely to be faithful?

The contrasts between selecting a leader and selecting a mate are instructive. Some dimensions of individual differences are critical to both decisions, such as differences in intelligence, honesty, and values. Other dimensions, however, are relevant to one sort of selection but irrelevant to the other. Differences in international clout may be critical to selecting a president, but irrelevant to selecting a mate. Differences in sexual adeptness may be critical to selecting a mate, but largely irrelevant to selecting a president.

The key point is that individual differences cannot be designated as "important" or "trivial" except with reference to some criterion. The criterion, in these examples, is which differences are relevant to solving the adaptive problem imposed by the selection being made. And because the individual differences that are critical *vary* depending on which adaptive problem one is confronting, it is always necessary to pose the question—Important for what purpose?

From an evolutionary psychological perspective, a sensible criterion for identifying *important* dimensions of individual differences is to examine our evolved psychological mechanisms for solving adaptive problems. Humans differ in an infinite number of ways. The differences that are important, however, are those that are linked with solving adaptive problems—that is, those linked with function. Over evolutionary time, those individuals who attended to and acted on individual differences in others that were adaptively consequential would have survived and reproduced more successfully than those who were oblivious to adaptively consequential differences in others. People who ignored individual differences in honesty, other things being equal, would have made poorer selections of mates and leaders than those who attended to, and acted on, these differences.

At this moment in time, all of us are the descendants of a long and unbroken line of ancestors who successfully solved the many complex problems entailed by survival and reproduction. As descendants of these successful ancestors, we carry with us the *difference-detecting mechanisms* that facilitated successful adaptive solutions. In order to understand what these difference-detecting mechanisms are, we must enter the minds of the individual problem solvers looking out at the social world inhabited by other individuals who differ in a bewildering variety of ways. We must enter the psychological mechanisms of the individual and ask two key questions: Which adaptive problem is the individual trying to solve? And which differences in other people are most relevant to solving, or failing to solve, these adaptive problems?

Strategic Interference and Strategic Facilitation

Our fears of snakes, spiders, heights, darkness, and strangers are elements in our strategies for survival. Our preferences for fat, sugar, salt, and protein are elements in our strategies for survival. Our blood-clotting mechanisms, callus-producing mechanisms, and tanning mechanisms are all elements in our strategies for survival.

Similarly, our preferences for particular mates are elements in our strategies for reproduction. Our emotion of jealousy is part gy for successful reproduction, because it functions productively relevant resources offered by a particu-y, Wilson, & Weghorst, 1982). None of these strate-_____ ᴜᴄ consciously articulated, of course, and most are not. When we consume a delicious dinner, we do not think to ourselves, "I am eating this meal because of the nutritive logic contained in the potassium, magnesium, and caloric properties that facilitate my bodily functioning and hence my survival." We simply get hungry, and certain foods taste great. Similarly, when we become attracted to a potential mate, we do not say to ourselves: "The selection of this mate will solve specific reproductive problems, and hence will increase my gene replication compared with alternative selections." We simply find ourselves mesmerized by some potential mates and indifferent to others. Our strategies, and the adaptive functions they were designed to serve, are largely outside of our conscious awareness.

Other individuals, however, can aid our solutions to adaptive problems or impede them. Just as eating a poisonous mushroom would interfere with our strategy for survival, selecting an unfaithful long-term mate would interfere with our strategy for reproduction. Just as selecting a habitat that offers water, ripe fruit, and shelter would facilitate our strategy for survival, selecting a mate who provides drink, food, and protection for our children would facilitate our strategy for reproduction.

We live in a social world, surrounded by other individuals who are pursuing their own strategies. Because evolution operates on a relative metric (*differential* reproductive success), the individuals who surround us are often competitors who are striving for precisely the same adaptively relevant resources. Good food, precious territory, elevated social status, powerful allies, and desirable mates are resources that are always in scarce supply compared with the numbers who seek them. One person's gain, therefore, often comes at the expense of others. In this sense, other individuals comprise our most important "hostile force of nature" (Alexander, 1987; Darwin, 1859).

An ancient Indian saying is that the only people who truly delight in your successes are your parents and your teachers (Devendra Singh, personal communication, June 1994). Hogan (Chapter 5, this volume) notes that elevated status often evokes the envy and resentment of others. Success and status are keenly sought but rarely attained. Just as our friends and loved ones help us with our strategies for getting ahead, our competitors collude to interfere with our strategies and tear us down. I call these phenomena *strategic facilitation* and *strategic interference,* respectively.

Strategic facilitation may be illustrated by a primate example. Among the chimpanzees, males vie for position as the dominant alpha male. Alpha status confers sexual access to mates. A typical alpha-male chimpanzee attains at least 50% of the copulations with females, and sometimes as many as 75% (de Waal, 1982). Peripheral low status males must settle for far fewer copulations and, in some cases, are literally banished from reproduction.

Given the reproductive benefits linked with alpha status, there is keen competition for position. A lone male, however, can rarely attain a dominant position without the aid of allies. In one study, the chimpanzee Yeroen, a formerly dominant male who had been ousted from power, formed an alliance with an upcoming male named Nikkie (de Waal, 1982). Although neither Yeroen nor Nikkie dared to challenge the dominant male Luit alone, together they made a formidable coalition. Over several weeks, the coalition grew bolder in challenging Luit. Eventually, a physical fight erupted. Although all the chimpanzees involved sustained injuries, the alliance of Nikkie and Yeroen triumphed. Following this victory, Nikkie secured 50% of the matings. But Yeroen, because of his alliance with Nikkie, now enjoyed 25% of the matings (up from 0%). Although he never again regained the dominant position, Yeroen had rallied from setback sufficiently to remain a contender in the troop.

This example illustrates one form of strategic facilitation. Yeroen and Nikkie, by selecting each other and forming a coalition, facilitated the success of both. The formation of alliances with others—friends, mates, or kin—is undoubtedly one of the most important means by which humans achieve their goals. Therefore, we would expect there to be tremendous evolutionary selection pressure for psychological mechanisms that guide the choices we make. We should have evolved preferences for allies who strategically facilitate our social goals, just as we have evolved preferences for foods that facilitate our survival goals. A guiding hypothesis of the evolutionary psychological perspective advanced here is that the dimensions of individual differences captured by the five-factor model are critical-selection dimensions for choosing allies who are strategic facilitators (Buss, 1989b).

The flip side of the coin to strategic facilitation is strategic interference. Some individuals impede our goals and block our strategies. Consider, for example, psychopathic individuals (Hare,

1993). Psychopaths typically exploit our cooperative mechanisms by appearing to be sound reciprocators. They gain our confidence by offering benefits at least commensurate with what they are getting from us. But over time, they defect. Psychopaths exploit the trust that they have gained to con us, often defecting on the last move of the social game. Successful psychopaths, in short, interfere with our strategy of forming successful reciprocal alliances.

In everyday social life, we are surrounded by a field of individuals, each of whom is pursuing an agenda and is carrying out strategies based on that agenda. Some of these individuals become allies with whom we join forces in strategic cooperation. Others interfere with our strategies and impede progress toward our goals and become our rivals and enemies. A guiding evolutionary hypothesis is that the dimensions captured by the five-factor model identify in broad brush strokes some of the most important costs and benefits linked with those who form our social adaptive landscape.

The Role of the Five Factors in Forming Strategic Alliances

As part of a larger study, Todd Dekay and I were interested in discovering how important each of the five factors is in forming different sorts of alliances with others (DeKay & Buss, in preparation). We focused on what we believe to be the three most important alliances we form with non-kin: *coalitions* (groups of individuals formed to achieve a common goal), *friendships* (dyadic reciprocal alliances), and *mateships* (long-term heterosexual alliances).

We asked subjects to judge each of 149 characteristics on how desirable or undesirable it was in a coalition partner, a friend, and a mate. Included within the 149 characteristics were markers of the five-factor model, selected on the basis of factor analyses reported by Goldberg (1983) and supplemented with evolutionarily guided markers. For *Surgency*, for example, we used dominant, bold, brave in the face of danger, and submissive. For *Agreeableness*, we used agreeable, kind, helpful to friends, and disagreeable. For *Conscientiousness*, we used hardworking, dependable, unreliable, and acting irresponsibly. For *Emotional Stability*, we used emotionally stable, emotionally unstable, and inability to handle stress well. For *Intellect–Openness*, we used intelligent, open-minded, stupid, and close-minded.

It is clear that the five factors figure prominently in all three forms of strategic alliance. When we examined the "top 20" most desirable characteristics out of the 149 characteristics in each of the three types of relationships, markers of the five factors appeared prominently in each. For *coalitions,* the following markers appeared in the most desirable 20: ambitious, bold, self-confident, and an exceptional leader (Surgency); kind (Agreeableness); hardworking and dependable (Conscientiousness); emotionally stable (Emotional Stability); and intelligent, open-minded, and having a wide range of knowledge (Intellect–Openness).

For *long-term mateships,* the following markers appeared among the most desirable 20 out of the 149 characteristics examined: self-confident, and ambitious about career goals (Surgency); kind (Agreeableness); dependable and hardworking (Conscientiousness); emotionally stable (Emotional Stability); intelligent, open-minded, and creative, with a wide range of knowledge (Intellect–Openness).

For *friendships,* the following markers appeared among the 20 most desirable characteristics out of the 149 attributes examined: bold, self-confident, and ambitious about career goals (Surgency); kind (Agreeableness); hardworking and dependable (Conscientiousness); emotionally stable (Emotional Stability); open-minded, intelligent, and creative, with a wide range of knowledge (Intellect–Openness).

It is clear that the individual differences captured by the five-factor model figure highly in desirable features of the major non-kin strategic relationships that men and women form in everyday life. In my view, these five factors are so important because they transcend relationship type; that is, Agreeableness, which signals (among other things) cooperativeness and a proclivity to be a good reciprocator, is critical for friendships, mateships, and coalitions. Conscientiousness, which signals dependability and industry, is also a valuable quality in each of the three types of relationships.

The foregoing does not imply that there are not important shifts in which individual differences are important in the different relationships. We found, for example, that being sexually unfaithful while in a steady relationship is viewed as mildly undesirable in a coalition member, moderately undesirable in a close friend, and extremely undesirable in a mateship. Similarly, kindness (Agreeableness) is judged to be more desirable in a mate than in a coalition member. The evolutionary psychological perspective expects some degree of domain specificity, because the precise individual differences that are important vary across different adaptive problems, and selecting a mate as opposed to a friend certainly constitutes distinct adaptive problems. Despite some degree of domain-specificity, the five factors of personality may be viewed as so important because their breadth allows them to transcend the particulars of specific relationships.

In summary, we have evidence that the individual differences captured by the five factors of personality are viewed as critical in forming strategic alliances of friendships, mateships, and coalitions. Are they also linked with aspects of strategic interference?

The Role of the Five Factors in Strategic Interference

If one end of each of the five factors is seen as desirable in strategic alliances, then the opposite end of each dimension should be linked with strategic interference. Although the empirical documentation of this proposition is incomplete, there is some evidence for it in the context of married couples (Buss, 1991a).

The five factors were assessed using a modification of an instrument developed by Goldberg (1983) and employing parallel forms in three data sources: self-report, spouse report, and interviewer reports (one male and one female interviewer, subsequently composited). Independently, members of married couples completed a 147-item instrument that assessed "Sources of Irritation and Upset" in the marriage. In particular, it provided a reasonably comprehensive assessment of the perceived costs that one's spouse inflicted, on the assumption that anger, irritation, and upset are emotions that signal strategic interference (Buss, 1989c).

By far the worst single source of anger and upset (strategic interference) was having a spouse who is *low on agreeableness*. Disagreeableness in spouses, as assessed via the three data sources, is linked with reports of neglect, verbal abuse, physical abuse, sexual infidelity, inconsiderateness, and self-centeredness. These results dovetail precisely with the expressed preferences in a mate—being kind topped the list of 149 attributes judged for desirability in a long-term mate (DeKay & Buss, in preparation). Interestingly, "Kind and Understanding" also received the top ranking of 13 characteristics ranked by 10,047 individuals from 37 cultures (Buss et al., 1990).

The second worst personality characteristic to have in a mate was *Emotional Instability*. Emotional Instability is linked with complaints by the spouse of being possessive, jealous, dependent, abusive, inconsiderate, physically self-absorbed, and self-centered. The other three dimensions are also linked with sources of upset. Low Conscientiousness is linked with sexual infidelity, particularly among men. Low Intellect–Openness is linked with the sexualizing of others (e.g., treating members of the opposite sex as sex objects; commenting about the attractiveness of others; expressing sexual desire for a movie star). And Surgency is linked with condescending actions, such as treating the spouse as inferior, placing more value on one's own opinions than on those of the spouse, and trying to act like he or she is better than the spouse.

In summary, this study provides promising evidence for links between the five factors of personality and sources of strategic interference. In the mating context, at least, it provides a detailed portrait of precisely what sorts of costs mates inflict on each other and, hence, the consequences of making a poor mate selection on the major dimensions of personality.

These preliminary studies suggest that the personality dimensions subsumed by the five-factor model are critically linked with strategic facilitation and strategic interference. The DeKay and Buss (in preparation) study shows that men and women alike value aspects of Surgency, Agreeableness, Conscientiousness, Emotional Stability, and Intellect–Openness in the social relations they form. Moreover, these valuable qualities appear to transcend relationship type; they are valued in long-term mates, in friends, and among coalition members. These personality factors, in short, appear to be important in establishing strategic alliances with others.

The five factors also are linked with various forms of strategic interference. In the study of married couples, spouses who are low on agreeableness and low on emotional stability seem especially problematical. Such persons are more likely to abuse their spouses verbally and physically. They are more likely to inflict damage by being sexually unfaithful. The five factors of personality, in short, appear to play a key role in strategic interference as well as in strategic facilitation.

Given the strategic import of the five factors of personality for critical selections, such as mate selection and friend selection, it would be astonishing if we found that men and women were passive with respect to communicating this information to others. To the contrary, the evolutionary psychological perspective proposed here suggests that the five factors would be targets in *strategic trait usage*

(Buss, 1989b). In other words, trait terms that signify standing on the five factors are predicted to be strategically applied to the self and to others in everyday usage in order to influence and manipulate the impressions that others form in order to accomplish adaptively significant goals. For example, they might be used to elevate one's own desirability (tactics of attraction) or to lower the desirability of rivals (derogation of competitors).

The Role of the Five Factors in Solving Adaptive Problems

Some individuals experience *greater success* at pursuing certain strategies rather than others: "Selection operates through the achievement of adaptive goal states, and any feature of the world—either of the environment, *or of one's own individual characteristics*—that influences the achievement of the relevant goal state may be assessed by an adaptively designed system" (Tooby & Cosmides, 1990, p. 59, italics added). Individuals who are mesomorphic, for example, typically will experience far greater success at enacting an aggressive strategy than individuals who are ectomorphic (Tooby & Cosmides call this phenomenon "reactive heritability").

Individual differences in physical attractiveness provide another example. There is evidence that physically attractive men are better able to successfully pursue a "short-term" mating strategy involving many sexual partners (Gangestad & Simpson, 1990). Physically attractive women are better able to pursue a long-term strategy of seeking and actually obtaining higher status higher income marriage partners (Taylor & Glenn, 1976). Relative physical attractiveness functions as "input" into species-typical or sex-typical psychological mechanisms, which then canalize the strategic solutions of different individuals in different directions.

The personality characteristics represented by the "Big Five" may represent (in part) individual differences in the qualities or resources individuals can draw upon to solve adaptive problems. The individual high on Surgency may be able to deploy socially dominant solutions. The person high on Agreeableness may be successful at eliciting cooperation from others in solving adaptive problems. The highly Conscientious person may solve adaptive problems through discipline, industry, and sheer hard work. The Emotionally Stable person may rely on steadiness of nerves, inner resiliency, and the capacity to rally from setback to solve adaptive problems. The person high on Intellectance may be adept at deploying creative cognitive solutions to adaptive problems.

In summary, this framework proposes a key role of personality in creating and solving adaptive problems:

1. Personality characteristics can play a causal role in determining the adaptive problems to which one is exposed.
2. The personality characteristics of people inhabiting one's social environment can play a causal role in imposing particular problems.
3. Personality characteristics influence the strategic solutions that people deploy to solve adaptive problems they confront.

An Illustration Using the Adaptive Problem of Spousal Infidelity

The Role of Personality in Creating Adaptive Problems

To examine the role of personality in the creation of adaptive problems, I conducted a longitudinal study of 100 married couples. During their newlywed year, we assessed the five major factors of personality through parallel instruments from three data sources—self-report, spouse-report, and independent-interviewer reports. Four years later, subjects completed a battery of instruments, including "Sources of Irritation and Upset," which contained 147 previously nominated things that a member of the opposite sex could do that might irritate, anger, annoy, or upset someone. Previous factor analyses of this instrument yielded 15 major sources of problems, including a cluster labeled "Infidelity." The Infidelity factor contained the following related complaints: "He or she saw someone else intimately"; "He or she had sex with another person"; "He or she was unfaithful to me"; "He or she went out with another person."

Low Conscientious men and women, as predicted, tend to inflict this adaptive problem on their spouses more than men and women higher in Conscientiousness. An unexpected finding was that women high on Intellect–Openness tended to inflict infidelity on their spouses. Personality of the spouse was also linked with the creation of problems other than infidelity, such as abuse, insults, neglect, and inconsiderateness. These results suggest that the personality characteristics of significant others inhabiting one's social milieu play a key role in creating adaptive problems.

Are some people exposed to the problem of spousal infidelity because of their own personality? To answer this question, we correlated personality characteristics of persons with the degree to which they complained about spousal infidelity. *Submissive* men and women—those low on Surgency—tended to complain that their spouses were unfaithful more than those higher on Surgency. Although correlational, these findings suggest that submissive people may be more at risk for encountering the problem of spousal infidelity; and marrying a mate low on Conscientiousness may put one at risk for incurring this adaptive problem.

The Role of Personality in Solving Adaptive Problems

Previous research has identified 19 distinct tactics that people use to retain their mates—tactics ranging from *vigilance* (e.g., "He kept a close eye on her at the party") to *violence* (e.g., "He hit a rival who was making moves on her"; Buss, 1988). We assessed the use of these tactics in the same sample of couples at two time periods (newlywed year and fourth year of marriage) using two data sources (self-report and spouse-report).

Men high on Surgency tend to retain their wives by frequent acts of *Resource Display* (e.g., "He spent a lot of money on her"; "He bought her an expensive gift"; "He took her out to a nice restaurant"). Men low on Surgency tended to use *Debasement* as a mate-retention tactic (e.g., "He told her that he would change in order to please her"; "He became a 'slave' to her"; "He gave in to her every wish"). Men high on Agreeableness tend to *Display Love and Care* (e.g., "He told her that he loved her"; "He went out of his way to be kind, nice, and caring"; "He was helpful when she really needed it"). In contrast, men low on Agreeableness tended to *Derogate Their Mate* (e.g., "He told other guys terrible things about her so that they wouldn't like her"; "He told other guys that she was not a nice person"; "He told other guys that she was stupid").

Men low on Conscientiousness tend to *Threaten Infidelity* (e.g., "He flirted with another woman in front of her"; "He went out with other women to make her jealous"). Men low on Emotional Stability tend to *Derogate Competitors* (e.g., "He cut down the appearance of other males"; "He told her the other guy was stupid"). Men low on

Intellect–Openness tend to *Threaten Violence* (e.g., "He yelled at other guys who looked at her"; "He stared coldly at the other guy who was looking at her"; "He threatened to hit the guy who was making moves on her").

These findings suggest that personality characteristics described by the Big Five are linked with the alternative tactics that men use to solve the problem of mate retention. Personality traits, as traditionally assessed, are linked in coherent ways with the tactics people use to accomplish goals and solve adaptive problems. An essential part of personality, in other words, consists of the recurrent strategies people use to solve adaptive problems.

Trait Usage as Manipulation

Over the past century, the dominant view of animal signals has been that their primary function is to facilitate communication between cooperative members of a species (Dawkins & Krebs, 1978; Parker, 1985). On this account, signals are designed to provide accurate information to others. Recent work in evolutionary biology suggests a less benevolent view. Animal signals generally, and human language specifically, may be viewed as evolved forms of manipulation that exploit the sense organs and behavioral machinery of others (Dawkins & Krebs, 1978; Krebs & Dawkins, 1984).

The display of anger, for example, rather than functioning to inform others about an internal state, may instead function to manipulate others to back down or to make threats more credible (Hirshleifer, 1987). Calling oneself smart or a competitor stupid may be designed to influence the impressions that others form, rather than to convey accurate information. We intuitively accept this view in the context of advertising and salesmanship. Advertisements are designed to persuade, not to inform. Dawkins and Krebs (1978) argue that this manipulative function is characteristic of communication generally.

This challenge to the "classical" view of language points to an important theoretical and empirical agenda—to chart the ways in which language is used by humans to achieve proximate goals that historically have been linked with reproductive success (Buss, 1986). The frequency and pervasiveness of trait-descriptive terms in the natural language suggest that this important agenda must be faced by personality psychologists. Personality language cannot be understood without understanding the *strategic functions* that its application serves for users in everyday life.

This view of trait usage does not imply deception and manipulation in all contexts. Evolutionary thinking provides instead a precise set of predictions about which contexts will involve accurate information transfer and which will involve deception. Trait usage should convey more accurate information to the extent that the adaptive interests of two interacting individuals coincide. To the extent that the interests of two individuals depart, then trait usage should depart from accurate information transfer.

Consider an illustration. If two men are both competing for sexual access to the same highly attractive woman, their goals conflict. In this context, an evolutionary psychological prediction is that these men will *exaggerate* their own positive traits in self-presentation to the woman, striving to appear to fulfill the characteristics that she desires in a mate. They will also *derogate* their competitor by exaggerating his negative traits, striving to portray the competitor as failing to embody or fulfill the characteristics that the woman desires in a mate. The brother or father of the woman, however, might convey to her *accurate* trait portraits of both male competitors; their adaptive interests, in this context, are more likely to coincide with hers.

In summary, there is no reason to assume that trait usage will be uniformly veridical in conveying accurate information. Indeed, we expect, on theoretical grounds, that trait usage, while always strategic and in that sense manipulative, can be either deceptive or accurate, depending on the context. Trait portrayal of the self and of others, therefore, should depend critically on the *goals* that humans are trying to achieve, on the *context* of surrounding conflicts and confluences of interests, and on the *strategies* that are deployed.

Trait Usage in Mate Attraction and Competitor Derogation

Sexual selection theory provides a powerful model for predicting forms of intrasexual competition. Competition for mates will center on embodying and displaying those characteristics that are desired by the opposite sex. In addition to predicting patterns of self-enhancement, analogous predictions can be made about patterns of derogation of competitors. Competitors will be derogated on those characteristics that the other sex desires.

Applying this model to the trait domain generates specific predictions, given our knowledge about what personality characteristics are desired in potential mates. Tactics to attract a mate should involved displaying Surgency, Agreeableness, Conscientiousness, Emotional Stability, and Intellect–Openness. Tactics to derogate intrasexual competitors should involve implying or demonstrating that the competitor is submissive (desurgent), disagreeable, unconscientious, emotionally unstable, and stupid.

Furthermore, because women value surgency or dominance in potential mates more than men do (Buss, 1989a, 1989b; Sadalla, Kenrick, & Vershure, 1987), it was predicted that men more than women will try to enhance their own surgency impressions when attempting to attract a mate; and that men more than women will try to derogate a competitor's surgency to make that competitor less desirable to the other sex. Men's tactics of trait manipulation, more than women's tactics, will center on this first factor of the five-factor model.

These predictions were generally confirmed in two empirical studies (Buss, 1989b). Men more than women mention their importance at work, boast about their accomplishments, and highlight their future ascendance in the hierarchy as part of their mate-attraction strategy. Furthermore, both sexes use tactics designed to appear *agreeable,* such as being sympathetic and helpful; *conscientious,* such as being well groomed and well mannered; and *intelligent,* such as acting sophisticated and displaying knowledge, vocabulary, and humor. No attraction tactics, however, appeared to involve signaling emotional stability.

Trait manipulation also figured prominently in tactics used to derogate competitors (Buss & Dedden, 1990). Men especially attempt to make their competitors appear to be lacking in surgency. They use tactics such as dominating their rival, mentioning that their rival lacks ambition, and asserting that the rival is cowardly, weak, and wimpy.

The low ends of each of the five factors are well represented in derogation tactics. Competitors are derogated by making them appear *disagreeable* (e.g., by calling them selfish, insensitive, inconsiderate, and self-centered); *unconscientious* (e.g., by calling them undisciplined, loose, cheating, and unclean); *emotionally unstable* (e.g., by saying that they are flighty and prone to crying); and *low on intellect* (e.g., by describing them as dumb, stupid, boring, uninteresting, and an airhead). The five factors of personality, in summary, figure prominently in the tactics that competitors use for the goal of denigrating their rivals.

Links between Evolutionary
and Other Theoretical Perspectives

In this section, I comment on the links between the current evolutionary psychological perspective and alternative theoretical perspectives on the five-factor model.

Hogan's Socioanalytic Theory

The evolutionary psychological perspective articulated here accords with Hogan's socioanalytic theory on several key assumptions. Both perspectives assume that human personality is best understood in the context of human evolution. Both perspectives take adaptation as critical, and view adaptations as products of evolution by selection. Both perspectives view group living as one of the most important "evolutionary environments" to which humans adapted. Both perspectives endorse a distinction between personality from the perspective of the actor versus personality from the perspective of the observer. And both perspectives stress human adaptations to group living, including *forming cooperative alliances* with others (Hogan's "getting along") and *negotiating hierarchies* (Hogan's "getting ahead") as defining features of human personality. In the conceptual space of all perspectives on personality, evolutionary psychology and socioanalytic theory are close; no other current theories take evolution and adaptation as essential foundations.

Despite broad-brush stroke similarities, the perspectives depart on several critical issues. One difference is the assumption about the number of evolved psychological mechanisms. Hogan (Chapter 5, this volume) assumes "a small number of unconscious biological needs." Evolutionary psychology, in contrast, emphasizes that humans have evolved an extraordinarily *large* number of psychological mechanisms, because the number of adaptive problems that humans have had to solve is very large. Thus, we are motivated not merely to "get along and get ahead," but also to select particular mates, particular friends, and particular coalitions (DeKay & Buss, in preparation); to ensure sexual fidelity and resource provisioning of mates, and continued reciprocity of friends (Buss, Larsen, Westen, & Semmelroth, 1992; Daly et al., 1982; Symons, 1979); to be sensitive to "cheating" in reciprocal relationships (Cosmides, 1989); to derogate our closest competitors (Buss & Dedden, 1990); and to solve a host of other social adaptive problems (Buss, 1994).

Although solving these numerous adaptive problems historically led to relatively greater survival and reproduction (and hence evolution of particular adaptive mechanisms), the evolved mechanisms cannot be "reduced" to a small number of "biological needs." Instantiated in our evolved brains and expressed through our evolved psychology are a large number of complex psychological mechanisms.

A second difference between the two perspectives is that whereas socioanalytic theory distinguishes between "actor" and "observer," evolutionary psychology partitions both into several separate analytic perspectives. An actor, for example, might display kindness toward a mate, ruthlessness toward an enemy, surgency toward a competitor, openness toward a child, and deference toward the "head man" in the tribe. From an observer's perspective, it matters a great deal whether the observer is an ally, a member of one's coalition, an enemy, or one's father. The personality features that are perceived, emphasized, and communicated to others in everyday life will depend in part on which of these numerous observer perspectives one takes, coupled with the degree to which the observer is at "strategic confluence" or "strategic interference" with the actor. Thus, although evolutionary psychology endorses Hogan's partition of actor and observer, it argues that Hogan does not go far enough in making important *perspectival distinctions.*

In summary, evolutionary psychology and socioanalytic theory are quite compatible with each other. Indeed, socioanalytic theory can be viewed as providing a powerful starting point for the evolutionary analysis of human personality. Evolutionary psychology adopts the evolutionary starting point of socioanalytic theory and expands it to account for the many complex adaptive problems humans confront, the numerous psychological mechanisms that comprise our solutions to those problems, and the critical perspectival differences inherent in social interaction.

McCrae and Costa's Dispositional Theory

McCrae and Costa (Chapter 3, this volume) assume that our basic psychological mechanisms evolved by a process of natural selection. It is now recognized that evolution occurs by a process of *differential reproductive success by virtue of heritable differences in design* (Williams, 1966; Symons, 1992). Hence, individuals are integrated collections of evolved adaptations. These collections are the "vehicles" by which gene replicators get transmitted to future generations.

McCrae and Costa focus their theory, however, not on universal aspects of personality, but on "personality-related individual differences in adaptation" (p. 32). As such, their theory is highly congruent with the evolutionary psychological formulation articulated here, which focuses on individual differences in the adaptive problems to which people are exposed and on individual differences in the ways in which people solve those adaptive problems. Furthermore, the two theoretical perspectives are in accord on viewing the five factors as capturing critical, adaptively relevant features of personality.

The two perspectives differ, however, on several key issues. The first stems from differences in whether universal aspects of human evolved psychology must be characterized in order to have a viable theory of individual differences. McCrae and Costa's position on this is: "To all such questions about the nature of human nature, trait psychology offers a single yet powerful answer: It varies" (p. 11). Furthermore, "the [five-factor trait] theory ignores universal aspects of personality . . . at the level of basic tendencies" (p. 32). The position of the evolutionary psychological perspective, however, is that one cannot understand individual variation without understanding the "universal design" that provides the parameters upon which variation can occur. Just as one cannot have a theory of "individual differences in cars" (e.g., variations in size, torque, horsepower, braking ability) without understanding "basic car mechanisms," one cannot have a theory of individual personality differences without understanding the common human psychology that forms the foundation upon which those differences are built.

A second critical difference is that McCrae and Costa (Chapter 3, this volume) do not explicitly define what they mean by "adaptation" or "individual differences in adaptation." The concept of "adaptation," however, is too critical to be left undefined or left to people's intuitions, which usually contain vague understandings about "the good of the person" or "the good of society." In the evolutionary psychological framework, adaptations are evolved solutions to problems of individual survival and reproduction. Individuals differ in many respects, including which adaptive problems they confront and which adaptive solutions they pursue.

In summary, the current proposal argues that human nature

cannot be ignored, but must instead form the backbone of a theory of personality, including a formulation of individual differences. Although the McCrae–Costa formulation and the current formulation concur that individual differences entail differences in adaptation, evolutionary psychology makes the concept of adaptation explicit and specifies several different routes by which individuals differ in adaptively relevant contexts.

Wiggins's Dyadic–Interactional Theory

The evolutionary psychological perspective accords with Wiggins's theory of dyadic exchanges in several key areas. Wiggins (1979, Chapter 4, this volume) argues that interpersonal transactions entail the exchange of love and status. Thus, the basic dimensions of personality flow from differences in these two forms of exchange. Surgency or dominance captures exchanges based on status. Agreeableness–quarrelsomeness captures exchanges based on love.

A key issue is: *Why* should exchanges of status and love be so central to human interaction? An evolutionary psychological perspective provides a powerful guide for determining why these transactions are so important. Among humans, reproductively relevant resources are closely linked with position in the status hierarchy. Among tribal societies, those of elevated status gain greater access to better food and territory. Elevated status also carries with it greater health care from others, especially for one's children (Hill & Hurtado, 1989). And not coincidentally, elevated status is closely linked with greater sexual access to more numerous mates for men in polygynous societies and access to more desirable mates for both women and men in presumptively monogamous societies (Buss, 1994).

Exchanges of love and hate are central to the issues of *strategic facilitation* and *strategic interference*. Positive affect flows to our mates, our friends, our coalitions, and our kin—those with whom we form strategic alliances. Negative affect flows toward those with whom we are at strategic interference—our competitors, rivals, and enemies (and sometimes to our mates and friends, when they impede our goals or frustrate our desires). Strategic alliances have always been critical to human survival and reproduction. Strategic interference has always been critical to impeding our survival and reproduction—other humans, in short, are our primary "hostile force of nature"

(Alexander, 1987). Exchanges of love and hate are important precisely because they signal these adaptive social problems.

Goldberg's Lexical Approach

The lexical approach of Goldberg (1981) starts with the assumption that the most significant individual differences in everyday-life interactions with others eventually become encoded as trait terms within the natural language. Presumably, these individual differences are critical in communicating with others, because language is a social medium.

Furthermore, Goldberg (1981) assumes that the five factors that emerge from the lexical approach are critical to answering questions that might be posed about a stranger with whom one might interact:

1. Is X active and dominant or passive and submissive? (Can I bully X or will X try to bully me?)
2. Is X agreeable (warm and pleasant) or disagreeable (cold and distant)?
3. Can I count on X? *(Is X responsible and conscientious or undependable and negligent?)*
4. Is X crazy (unpredictable) or sane (stable)?
5. Is X smart or dumb? (How easy will it be for me to teach X?)

By posing these questions, Goldberg pointed to an important agenda for the field of personality: What information does trait usage convey that is critical to interacting with others in everyday life?

Evolutionary psychology provides a *heuristic* for addressing this critical question. We might reformulate Goldberg's questions by infusing them with adaptively relevant content:

1. How powerful is X and where is he or she in the status hierarchy (Surgency–Submissivness)?
2. Is this person a strategic cooperator or will he or she interfere with the pursuit of my strategies (Agreeableness–Quarrelsomeness)?
3. Can this person be trusted, or will he or she defect (Conscientiousness–Unreliability)?
4. Is this person in command of his or her personal resources,

or does he or she have a volatile and tenuous hold on them (Emotional Stability–Emotional Instability)?

5. At what level should I pitch my attempts at strategic manipulation (Intellect–Openness vs. Stupidity–Boorishness)?

Is the Five-Factor Model Comprehensive from an Evolutionary Psychological Perspective?

From the current theoretical perspective, it is unlikely that the five factors alone will prove to be sufficient. One reason for this view is that many important individual differences are not captured, or are only obliquely captured, by the five factors. One example will be used to illustrate this point—individual differences in sexuality.

In the history of the lexical approach that led to the five factors, several important exclusionary criteria were used to reduce the list of traits to a more manageable number. For example, words that tended to be "sex-linked" were excluded (Norman, 1967). Thus, individual differences in "coyness" were excluded because the term "coy" was presumed to be more relevant to women than to men. Unfortunately, *many* individual differences in the sexual sphere tend to be sex-linked in this manner. Thus, the use of "sex-linkage" as an exclusion criterion inadvertently resulted in the near total omission of individual differences in sexuality.

Recently, David Schmitt and I (Schmitt & Buss, under review) excavated all trait terms that referred to individual differences in sexuality—terms such as "coy," "chaste," "sexy," "promiscuous," and "prudish." Factor analyses of these terms, in conjunction with the five factors, revealed that although some dimensions of sexuality were correlated with the five factors, several of the sexuality dimensions contained substantial variance independent of the five-factor model. Furthermore, some individual differences in sexuality were orthogonal to the five factors and formed their own factors. Individual differences in sexuality are critical from an evolutionary perspective, because they signify differences in "sexual strategy" (Buss & Schmitt, 1993).

To say that the five factors are unlikely to be comprehensive in no way denies their profound significance. Indeed, a plausible argument can be made that the five factors capture individual differences that transcend a wide variety of social interactions, including mateships, friendships, kinships, and coalitions. In contrast, other differences—

such as differences in sexual strategy—become important in more narrowly delineated social contexts, such as mating. This merely highlights a central theme of this chapter: When posing the question of importance, it is critical to ask *important for what adaptive purpose?*

Discussion

The current chapter argues for extending the study of personality traits in two related directions. The first is understanding the role of personality traits in social interaction. The results of the study of personality and mate-retention tactics, for example, demonstrate clearly that personality traits such as Surgency, Agreeableness, and Conscientiousness have profound consequences for social behavior in the mating domain. Other studies have shown the importance of personality in social domains, such as the tactics people use to influence others (Buss, 1992), and conflict in married couples (Buss, 1991a). These efforts represent just the start of understanding the important role that personality traits play in social interaction.

The second new direction for personality, closely related to the first, is adding *functional analysis* to the understanding of personality traits. This level entails examining the role of personality traits in creating adaptive problems, and perhaps more important, the role of personality in solving adaptive problems. The finding that major traits such as Surgency, Agreeableness, and Emotional Stability are linked with the solutions individuals deploy to solve the problem of mate retention provides just one illustration of this new level of analysis.

By adding these related levels of analysis to our field, we elevate the study of personality traits to a more important place within the broader field of psychology. Personality psychology is now poised to expand beyond the province of a small group of technical specialists. Personality traits play a major role in the central concerns of other branches of psychology, such as social psychology and developmental psychology. And the evolutionary psychology framework demonstrates that personality traits are not isolated from the universal human mechanisms that form the core of other branches of psychology. Personality traits and universal psychological mechanisms can be integrated within a single, unified conceptual framework. Theoretical perspectives on the five-factor model provide an important step toward this integrative direction.

Acknowledgments

I thank Todd DeKay, Heidi Greiling, Robert Hogan, Jeff McCrae, Todd Shackelford, and Jerry Wiggins for helpful comments on earlier drafts of this chapter.

References

Alexander, R. D. (1987). *The biology of moral systems.* New York: deGruyter.

Block, J. (1995). A contrarian view of the five-factor approach to personality description. *Psychological Bulletin, 117,* 187–215.

Buss, D. M. (1986). Can social science be anchored in evolutionary biology? *Revue Européene des Sciences Sociales, 24,* 41–50.

Buss, D. M. (1988). From vigilance to violence: Mate retention tactics. *Ethology and Sociobiology, 9,* 291–317.

Buss, D. M. (1989a). Sex differences in mate preferences: Evolutionary hypotheses tested in 37 cultures. *Behavioral and Brain Sciences, 12,* 1–49.

Buss, D. M. (1989b, June). *A theory of strategic trait usage: Personality and the adaptive landscape.* Paper presented at the Invited Workshop on Personality Language, University of Groningen, The Netherlands.

Buss, D. M. (1989c). Conflict between the sexes: Strategic interference and the evocation of anger and upset. *Journal of Personality and Social Psychology, 56,* 735–747.

Buss, D. M. (1991a). Conflict in married couples: Personality predictors of anger and upset. *Journal of Personality, 59,* 663–688.

Buss, D. M. (1991b). Evolutionary personality psychology. *Annual Review of Psychology, 42,* 459–491.

Buss, D. M. (1992). Manipulation in close relationships: Five personality factors in interactional context. *Journal of Personality, 60,* 477–499.

Buss, D. M. (1994). *The evolution of desire: Strategies of human mating.* New York: Basic Books.

Buss, D. M. (1995). Evolutionary psychology: A new paradigm for psychological science. *Psychological Inquiry, 6,* 1–30.

Buss, D. M., Abbott, M., Angleitner, A., Asherian, A., Biaggio, A., et al. (1990). International preferences in mate selection. *Journal of Cross-Cultural Psychology, 21,* 5–47.

Buss, D. M., & Dedden, L. A. (1990). Derogation of competitors. *Journal of Social and Personal Relationships, 7,* 395–422.

Buss, D. M., Larsen, R., Westen, D., & Semmelroth, J. (1992). Sex differences in jealousy: Evolution, physiology, and psychology. *Psychological Science, 3,* 251–255.

Buss, D. M., & Schmitt, D. P. (1993). Sexual Strategies Theory: The evolutionary psychology of human mating. *Psychological Review, 100,* 204–232.

Cosmides, L. (1989). The logic of social exchange: Has natural selection shaped how humans reason? *Cognition, 31,* 187–276.

Daly, M., Wilson, M., & Weghorst, S. J. (1982). Male sexual jealousy. *Ethology and Sociobiology, 3,* 11–27.

Darwin, C. (1859). *On the origin of the species by means of natural selection, or Preservation of favoured races in the struggle for life.* London: Murray.

Dawkins, R., & Krebs, J. R. (1978). Animal signals: Information or manipulation? In J.R. Krebs & N.B. Davies (Eds.), *Behavioral ecology: An evolutionary approach* (pp. 282–309). Oxford: Blackwell.

DeKay, W. T., & Buss, D. M. (in preparation). *Desirable characteristics in mates, friends, and coalitions.*

de Waal, F. (1982). *Chimpanzee politics: Power and sex among the apes.* Baltimore: Johns Hopkins University Press.

Gangestad, S. W., & Simpson, J. A. (1990). Toward an evolutionary history of female sociosexual variation. *Journal of Personality, 58,* 69–96.

Goldberg, L. R. (1972). Some recent trends in personality assessment. *Journal of Personality Assessment, 36,* 547–560.

Goldberg, L. R. (1981). Language and individual differences: The search for universals in personality lexicons. In L. Wheeler (Ed.), *Review of personality and social psychology* (pp. 141–165). Beverly Hills, CA: Sage.

Goldberg, L. R. (1983, June). *The magical number five, plus or minus two: Some considerations on the dimensionality of personality descriptors.* Paper presented at a research seminar, Gerontology Research Center, National Institute on Aging/National Institutes of Health, Baltimore, MD.

Goldberg, L. R. (1992). The development of markers of the Big-Five factor structure. *Psychological Assessment, 4,* 26–42.

Hare, R. D. (1993). *Without conscience.* New York: Pocket Books.

Hill, K. & Hurtado, A. M. (1989). Hunter–gatherers of the new world. *American Scientist, 77,* 437–443.

Hirshleifer, J. (1987). On the emotions as guarantors of threats and promises. In J. Dupre (Ed.), *The latest on the best: Essays on evolutionary optimality* (pp. 277–306). Cambridge, MA: MIT Press.

Hofstee, W. K. B., De Raad, B., & Goldberg, L. R. (1992). Integration of the Big Five and circumplex approaches to trait structure. *Journal of Personality and Social Psychology, 63,* 146–163.

Hogan, R. (1983). A socioanalytic theory of personality. In M. M. Page (Ed.), *Personality: Current theory and research* (pp. 55–89). Lincoln: University of Nebraska Press.

John, O. P. (1990). The "Big-Five" factor taxonomy: Dimensions of personality in the natural language and in questionnaires. In L. Pervin (Ed.), *Handbook of personality: Theory and research* (pp. 66–100). New York: Guilford Press.

Krebs, J. R., & Dawkins, R. (1984). Animal signals: Mind-reading and manipulation. In J. R. Krebs & N. B. Davies (Eds.), *Behavioral ecology: An evolutionary approach* (2nd ed., pp. 380–402). Oxford: Blackwell.

Kyl-Heku, L., & Buss, D. M. (under review). *Tactics of hierarchy negotiation.*

McCrae, R. R., & John, O. P. (1992). An introduction to the five-factor model and its applications. *Journal of Personality, 60,* 175–215.

Norman, W. T. (1963). Toward an adequate taxonomy of personality attributes: Replicated factor structure in peer nomination personality ratings. *Journal of Abnormal and Social Psychology, 66,* 574–583.

Norman, W. T. (1967). *2800 personality trait descriptors: Normative operating characteristics for a university population.* Ann Arbor: Department of Psychology, University of Michigan.

Parker, S. T. (1985). A socio-technological model for the evolution of language. *Current Anthropology, 26,* 617–639.

Sadalla, E. K., Kenrick, D. T., & Vershure, B. (1987). Dominance and heterosexual attraction. *Journal of Personality and Social Psychology, 52,* 730–738.

Schmitt, D. P., & Buss, D. M. (under review). *Dimensions of individual differences in the sexual domain: Beyond or subsumed by the five-factor model?*

Stone, V. E. (1989). *Perception of status: An evolutionary analysis of nonverbal status cues.* Doctoral dissertation, Department of Psychology, Stanford University, Stanford, CA.

Symons, D. (1979). *The evolution of human sexuality.* New York: Oxford University Press.

Symons, D. (1992). On the use and misuse of Darwinism in the study of human behavior. In J. Barkow, L. Cosmides, & J. Tooby (Eds.), *The adapted mind* (pp. 137–159). New York: Oxford University Press.

Taylor, P. A., and Glenn, N. D. (1976). The utility of education and attractiveness for females' status attainment through marriage. *American Sociological Review, 41,* 484–498.

Tooby, J., & Cosmides, L. (1990). On the universality of human nature and the uniqueness of the individual: The role of genetics and adaptation. *Journal of Personality, 58,* 17–68.

Tooby, J., & Cosmides, L. (1992). Psychological foundations of culture. In J. Barkow, L. Cosmides, & J. Tooby (Eds.), *The adapted mind: Evolutionary psychology and the generation of culture* (pp. 19–136). New York: Oxford University Press.

Waller, N. G., & Ben-Porath, Y. S. (1987). Is it time for clinical psychology to embrace the five-factor model of personality? *American Psychologist, 42,* 887–889.

Wiggins, J. S. (1979). A psychological taxonomy of trait descriptive terms: The interpersonal domain. *Journal of Personality and Social Psychology, 37,* 395–412.

Wiggins, J. S. (1991). Agency and communion as conceptual coordinates for the understanding and measurement of interpersonal behavior. In W. Grove & D. Cicchetti (Eds.), *Thinking clearly about psychology: Essays in honor of Paul E. Meehl* (Vol. 2, pp. 89–113). Minneapolis: University of Minnesota Press.

Wiggins, J. S., & Trapnell, P. D. (in press). Personality structure: The return of the Big Five. In R. Hogan, J. Johnson, & S. R. Briggs (Eds.), *Handbook of personality psychology.* Orlando, FL: Academic Press.

Williams, G. C. 1966. *Adaptation and natural selection.* Princeton, NJ: Princeton University Press.

Index

on Guilford and Guilford scale, 4
and marital fidelity, 193, 195
replicability of, 39–40
in solving adaptive problems, 193, 197
in strategic interference, 191
Intellectual perspectives, 14
Interdependence, 97
Interpersonal Adjectives Scales (IAS), 124–126, 128, 130–133, 145
revised, 63
Interpersonal Behavior Inventory, 132
Interpersonal processes, 63, 71, 100, 116–134, 165, 176, 203; *see also* Social exchange
field forces in, 117
measurement methods for, 129–130
measurement of variables in, 121–129
in psychotherapy, 116, 118–119
reciprocal patterns in, 116
and status/acceptance, 168
and unit of observation, 109, 120, 130
Interpersonal Style Inventory (ISI), 63
Intimacy, 98–100; *see also* Love
Introversion, 4
Inventory of Interpersonal Problems (IIP), 131–134

L

Language, 37, 90, 202; *see also* Lexical hypothesis
and communication, 34, 180, 202
and factor locations, 36
as manipulation, 195
and personality, 26–28, 33–34, 61
Leader selection, 184
Lexical hypothesis, 16*n*.1, 22–45, 61, 180, 202–203
and Big Five model, 36–43

continuum in, 38
as descriptive approach, 25
explications of, 23
and phenotypic attributes, 26
and real-world reference, 27, 34
universality in, 35–36
variables in, 28–29
Life course, 70, 74, 78
Life narrative, 69, 91, 97–100, 149*n*.2
nuclear episodes in, 99
Life Record (*L*-data), 2
Liking for Thinking, 4; *see also* Intellect (Openness) factor
Linguistic relativity, 27
Love, 98, 114
and anxiety, 112, 114
denying, 149*n*.3
and interpersonal variables, 121–125
as motivation, 99
as resource, 101–108, 201
Love Attitudes Scale, 139

M

Maladjustment, 74, 76
Manifest Anxiety scale, 138
Manipulation, 195–197
Masculinity versus femininity in factor conception, 9, 144
Mate selection, 92, 183–186, 188–191, 198, 204
and status, 201
trait usage in, 196
Maturity factor, 3
Memory, 175
Millon Clinical Multiaxial Inventory, 134
Minnesota Multiphasic Personality Inventory (MMPI), 127, 138–139, 141, 164
Personality Disorder scales, 63
Money, as resource, 101–108, 114
Mother–infant relationship, 110–111
Motivational tendencies, 63, 69, 105, 115, 220